MULTIPLE RELATION⬧ W9-BHM-737
CONFLICT OF INTEREST FOR
MENTAL HEALTH PROFESSIONALS

A Conservative Psycholegal Approach

Bruce W. Ebert, PhD, JD
Former Chair, California Board of Psychology

Professional Resource Press
Sarasota, Florida

Published by
Professional Resource Press
(An imprint of Professional Resource Exchange, Inc.)
Post Office Box 15560
Sarasota, FL 34277-1560

This publication is sold with the understanding that the Publisher is not engaged in rendering professional services. If legal, psychological, medical, accounting, or other expert advice or assistance is sought or required, the reader should seek the services of a competent professional.

The copy editor for this book was Patricia Rockwood, the managing editor was Debbie Fink, the production coordinator was Laurie Girsch, the typesetter was Richard Sullivan, and the cover designer was Krista Kauffman.

Library of Congress Cataloging-in-Publication Data

Ebert, Bruce W., date.
  Multiple relationships and conflict of interest for mental health professionals : a conservative psycholegal approach / Bruce W. Ebert.
     p. cm.
  Includes bibliographical references and index.
  ISBN 1-56887-098-1 (alk. paper)
     1. Mental health personnel and patient--Moral and ethical aspects. 2. Psychotherapist and patient--Moral and ethical aspects. 3. Mental health personnel--Legal status, laws, etc. 4. Mental health personnel--Professional ethics. 5. Mental health personnel--Sexual behavior. 6. Mental health personnel--Malpractice. 7. Sex between psychotherapist and patient. 8. Interpersonal relations. I. Title.

  RC480.8.E24 2006

  174.2'9689--dc22

                                                                                2005040186

ISBN-13: 978-1-56887-098-4
ISBN-10: 1-56887-098-1

DEDICATION

In Memoriam

Donald C. Ebert
1916 - 2004

ACKNOWLEDGMENTS

This has been a long-term project. In fact, this book has taken approximately 7 years to get to publication. Many individuals have played an important part in assisting me with the various aspects of this book. My deepest and most sincere thanks go to Dr. Larry Ritt, president of Professional Resource Press, who continuously believed in me through the ups and downs of writing this manuscript. His unyielding faith and positive comments have been critical to the fruition of this project. I also deeply appreciate Debra Fink, the managing editor for PRP, who worked tirelessly through numerous changes, making this book into something I am proud to have written and feel I would never have completed without her continuous help and willingness to take extensive time in reviewing and correcting the manuscript.

There are many others along the way who have helped me in the writing of this book. Tom O'Connor, former Executive Officer of the California Board of Psychology, requires credit for his help with identification of actual cases involving multiple role relationships during a time when I was an advocate/attorney, representing clients against the very Board of Psychology where he worked. Special thanks go to Dr. Marty Greenberg for our very thoughtful discussions and conversations over the years regarding ethical and legal issues. I am also extremely grateful to Eiran D. Mitchell, who provided a great deal of work typing, editing, and retyping copies of the manuscript, working tirelessly to assist me in getting the final product to publication. I am also very pleased to have had the opportunity to work with Dr. Ofer Zur and Dr. Arnold Lazarus. Although we differed in our opinions, they nevertheless provided an important perspective for me to rationally distinguish our thinking regarding multiple role relationships.

I am extremely grateful to my family, including my wife Pamela and younger daughter Ali, who gave up a great deal of family time while I was upstairs in my office, writing this book. I also want to thank my older daughter, Andrea, who spent many hours working with me, editing the manuscript and reading various versions of it to get it ready for publication. I am very appreciative to my whole family for their support and understanding during the writing of this book. Also many thanks to the numerous other people who, over the years, have aided me in the completion of this project.

TABLE OF CONTENTS

PREFACE

In this book I examine many cases dealing with multiple relationships, all of which were either charged by a licensing board or were part of a malpractice action or an ethics committee complaint. Although books and articles that offer alternative thinking about multiple relationships are an important contribution to the ongoing dialogue among mental health professionals regarding evolving standards of ethics, following the advice given in such publications may result in the loss of a license, imprisonment, expulsion from an organization, job action, civil suits, and removal from a managed care panel. The unique contribution of this book is to present a conservative approach to dealing with multiple relationship issues. Each chapter will identify a different issue and discuss the specific rules pertaining to that issue which are generally accepted in the licensing of a mental health professional. In addition, discussions of ethics and law, and areas of controversy, will be included. Use of this book will serve as a guide to limit clinicians' exposure to complaints. By following the guidelines in this book and learning from others' mistakes, the reader will mitigate risks and, thus, enjoy a lifelong practice. Throughout this book, the reader will learn the central idea that ethical practice is based upon a commitment to virtue which is applied to all aspects of professional practice.

— *Bruce W. Ebert*
Roseville, California
December 2005

MULTIPLE RELATIONSHIPS AND CONFLICT OF INTEREST FOR MENTAL HEALTH PROFESSIONALS

A Conservative Psycholegal Approach

MULTIPLE RELATIONSHIPS: BACKGROUND

In the movie *Antwone Fisher* (2002), which is based on a true story, actor Denzel Washington plays the role of a Navy psychiatrist who is both ethical and who goes far beyond what is required of him to assist a young seaman, Antwone Fisher, who is constantly in trouble because of his anger. His anger apparently stems, in part, from his lack of connection with his biological family. The Navy psychiatrist goes out of his way to assist Mr. Fisher by seeing him in his office, visiting him when he is in the brig, inviting him for dinner, and having numerous contacts with him outside of the confines of the therapy office. Although this might be seen as a demonstration of a multiple relationship, what makes this situation unique and acceptable is that the behavior exhibited by the Navy psychiatrist does not involve exploitation of his patient, he does not abuse his patient, he is not driven by self-interest, nor is the relationship designed to meet the exclusive needs of the psychiatrist, although some of his needs are met. The cases discussed in this book are opposite to that type of multiple relationship displayed in the story of *Antwone Fisher*. Because multiple relationships are so complex, it is important to understand the development of multiple relationship provisions before addressing specific issues.

In 1958, the American Psychological Association (APA) created a prohibition against providing treatment to clients when certain types of dual relationships existed (APA, 1958). In 1977, those dual relationships were prohibited if they were exploitative in nature (APA, 1977). The designation of dual relationships as an ethical problem appeared in the section of the ethics code entitled Welfare of the Consumer in 1977, but it was placed in a category called Client Relationship in 1958. The same language used in the 1977 ethics code appeared in the 1979 revision (APA, 1979). The primary reason to classify exploitative dual relationships as unethical was to attempt to prevent therapists from entering into clinical relationships where a prior relationship (e.g.,

1

family member, close friend) or new relationship (e.g., business partner, coworker) may interfere with the therapist's ability to provide objective treatment to the patient (APA, 1958). Later, the term gained recognition in its use essentially to prohibit therapists from engaging in sexual relations with their patients. It is interesting to note that the term was never used to preclude a therapist from establishing dual or multiple relationships after therapy began. Further, the term was exclusively applied to the provision of therapy and not to other professional services such as consultation, supervision, forensic practice, or in an evaluation scenario such as in a worker's compensation or Americans With Disabilities Act case. The development of ethical language on dual relationships has evolved through the years. Table 1 (pp. 6-8) compares the language in various ethics codes pertaining to dual relationships.*

Other professional ethics codes have been clearer and more explicit about their prohibitions of exploitative dual relationships (American Association for Marriage and Family Therapy [AAMFT], 2001). However, there were antecedent principles to the prohibitions on dual and multiple relationships proposed by professional groups, all of which dealt with preventing harm to a patient or preventing a loss of objectivity in the therapeutic relationship. The most modern language dealing with multiple relationships comes from the new code of ethics of the American Psychological Association (APA, 2002).

Not all multiple relationships are unethical. Although all major mental health professions have a prohibition against entering into multiple relationships that are harmful and/or exploitative to the client, the forgotten aspect of these prohibitions, in essence, is that only those multiple role relationships that are harmful to or against the interests of the client are prohibited. To date, within the United States, no professional association or licensing board has concluded that all multiple relationships are either unethical or illegal. Despite this, some licensing boards and ethics committees seem to approach ethical and licensing complaints with the misguided and erroneous idea that all multiple relationships are unethical or illegal.

The *Code of Ethics* of the American Association for Marriage and Family Therapy prohibits exploitative dual relationships. Principle 1.3 of the AAMFT *Code of Ethics* states: "Therapists, therefore, make every effort to avoid conditions and multiple relationships with clients that could impair professional judgment or increase the risk of exploitation." The National Association of Social Workers (NASW;

---

* See Appendix A (pp. 167-168) for a list of professional organizations that may be contacted to obtain complete copies of their codes of ethics.

1999) *Code of Ethics* does contain precise language which prohibits dual relationships. Standard 1.06(c), one of the provisions under the section "Conflicts of Interest," states: "Social workers should not engage in dual or multiple relationships with clients or former clients in which there is a risk of exploitation or potential harm to the client." All provisions in this section contain clear prohibitions against engaging in behavior that contravenes the interest of the client.

Similarly, psychiatrists are prohibited from exploiting their patients, but the terms "dual relationships" or "multiple relationships" are not present in *The Principles of Medical Ethics With Annotations Especially Applicable to Psychiatry* (American Psychiatric Association, 2001). Section 1(1) states: "A psychiatrist shall not gratify his or her own needs by exploiting the patient."

In Section A.5.c., the *ACA Code of Ethics* of the American Counseling Association (ACA, 2005) states:

> Counselor–client nonprofessional relationships with clients, former clients, their romantic partners, or their family members should be avoided, except when the interaction is potentially beneficial to the client. *(See A.5.d.)*

The American Association of Pastoral Counselors (AAPC), Principle III—Client Relationships, states:

> We avoid those dual relationships with clients (e.g., business or close personal relationships) which could impair our professional judgment, compromise the integrity of the treatment, and/or use the relationship for our own gain. (AAPC, 1994, Section III.E)

There is a coalescence of opinion among professional organizations regarding those multiple relationships that are unethical. During the past few years numerous articles have been written on the subject of dual relationships. These articles have provided significant advances in the conceptual understanding of dual relationship issues. Some authors have focused on state licensing board actions regarding dual relationships (Bader, 1994; Gottlieb, Sell, & Schoenfeld, 1988), some have explored general ethical issues (Youngren & Skorka, 1992), while others have identified unique problems such as avoiding dual relationships in a rural area (Jennings, 1992). Some have argued that the prohibitions against dual relationships have gone too far (Clarkson, 1994). It is clear that dual relationship problems are prevalent and present significant concerns for mental health professionals (Borys & Pope, 1989). Modern writers in the field of psychological ethics have written more extensively about the significant problems that can arise in multiple relationships (Bersoff, 2003; Knapp & VandeCreek, 2003; Lazarus & Zur, 2002; Syme, 2003). Unique problems in dual relationships arise in dealing with certain populations. An example of a case where a dual relationship is ethical and helpful to the client can be found in Cavallara and Ramsey's (1988) discussion of provision of services to geriatric patients.

There are clear cases where there is a dual relationship that is ethical and helpful to the client. However, in each of these cases there is no exploitation, harm, or damage to the client, and the focus is on assisting the client.

Mental health professionals need an analytical model to use in evaluating multiple relationships. The rules surrounding multiple relationships must be constitutionally sound and must protect the interests of the client, but must not be overly prohibitive to mental health professionals. Further, there is a need for a definitive work detailing the problems of multiple relationships and describing methods of resolving conflicts.

The problem is further complicated by the environment in which a mental health professional works. Those who are employed in rural settings, for example, constantly face multiple relationships with their clients. It would be fundamentally unfair to discipline a professional working in a rural setting for being involved in multiple relationships, depending, of course, upon the nature of such relationships. No one would condone sexual conduct with a client simply because it occurred in a rural setting. But would everyone universally conclude a mental health professional to be unethical who provides therapy (for a reasonable fee) to a local grocer in a rural town, where only one such store exists, unless there is direct evidence of exploitation? Would a psychologist who works in a community mental health center with seriously disturbed patients be labeled unethical for assisting them in participating in an onsite agency work project such as a community kitchen?* Would a social worker who is employed in Barrow, Alaska, be disciplined for accepting fish as payment where the exact value of the fish could not be determined? Multiple relationship issues present a significant problem to licensing boards as well as to professional associations. Consider the data gathered by the Association of State and Provincial Psychology Boards (ASPPB) over 20 years beginning in 1983, which is presented in Table 2 (p. 9).

---

* In Placer County, California, the County Mental Health Department has created a small restaurant, called Eleanor's Cupboard, which serves county workers. It is staffed by seriously mentally ill patients of the county mental health center and supervised by therapists working for the county. This is an example of a dual relationship, but how could this worthy effort be labeled as unethical?

Also consider data from the State of California Licensing Boards, the largest regulatory board of mental health professionals. Tables 3a and 3b (pp. 10-11) present this data.

Likewise, the National Organization of Licensing Boards in Social Work has compiled ethics data for the past 10 years. Those data are enlightening as well, and are presented in Table 4 (p. 12)

The data indicate that a dual relationship which includes sexual misconduct is a significant disciplinary problem for mental health professionals. There is a need for clear rules, clear prohibitions, and for mental health professionals to engage in safe practices. Also necessary is a method of conceptually analyzing multiple relationship issues. There are guiding ethical principles that are far more important than ubiquitous prohibitions for therapists, consultants, evaluators, and supervisors to follow in order to truly assist clients and other consumers who are in need of high-quality services from ethical professionals. Again, not all multiple relationships are unethical. Examples of unethical relationships would be those relationships that either cause or are likely to cause harm to the client, those that are likely to lead to exploitation, those that are not entered into with the client's best interest at heart, or those that would impair the objectivity of the professional providing mental health services. A relatively new movement called "virtue based ethics" should provide the foundation for mental health practice (E. D. Cohen & G. S. Cohen, 1999; Pettifor, 1996). Discussion of the role of virtue in ethics may be found in Chapter 13.

TABLE 1: Dual Relationship Ethics

American Psychological Association (APA)

§ 3.05   Multiple Relationships

(a) A multiple relationship occurs when a psychologist is in a professional role with a person and (1) at the same time is in another role with the same person, (2) at the same time is in a relationship with a person closely associated with or related to the person with whom the psychologist has the professional relationship, or (3) promises to enter into another relationship in the future with the person or a person closely associated with or related to the person.

A psychologist refrains from entering into a multiple relationship if the multiple relationship could reasonably be expected to impair the psychologist's objectivity, competence, or effectiveness in performing his or her functions as a psychologist, or otherwise risks exploitation or harm to the person with whom the professional relationship exists.

Multiple relationships that would not reasonably be expected to cause impairment or risk exploitation or harm are not unethical.

(b) If a psychologist finds that, due to unforeseen factors, a potentially harmful multiple relationship has arisen, the psychologist takes reasonable steps to resolve it with due regard for the best interests of the affected person and maximal compliance with the Ethics Code.

(c) When psychologists are required by law, institutional policy, or extraordinary circumstances to serve in more than one role in judicial or administrative proceedings, at the outset they clarify role expectations and the extent of confidentiality and thereafter as changes occur. (See also Standards 3.04, Avoiding Harm, and 3.07, Third-Party Requests for Services.)

American Association for Marriage and Family Therapy (AAMFT)

§ 1.3   Marriage and family therapists are aware of their influential positions with respect to clients, and they avoid exploiting the trust and dependency of such persons. Therapists, therefore, make every effort to avoid conditions and multiple relationships with clients that could impair professional judgment or increase risk of exploitation. Such dual relationships include, but are not limited to, business or close personal relationships with a client or the client's immediate family. When the risk of impairment or exploitation exists due to conditions or multiple roles, therapists take appropriate precautions.

§ 4.1   Marriage and Family therapists are aware of their influential positions with respect to students and supervisees, and they avoid exploiting the trust and dependency of such persons.

National Association of Social Workers (NASW)

§ 1.06(c) Social workers should not engage in dual or multiple relationships with clients or former clients in which there is a risk of exploitation or potential harm to the client.

American Psychiatric Association

§ 1.1 A psychiatrist should not gratify his or her own needs by exploiting the patient. The psychiatrist shall be ever vigilant about the impact that his or her conduct has upon the boundaries of the doctor–patient relationship, and thus upon the well-being of the patient. These requirements become particularly important because of the essentially private, highly personal, and sometimes intensely emotional nature of the relationship established with the psychiatrist.

American Counseling Association (ACA)

§ A.5.c. **Nonprofessional Interactions or Relationships (Other Than Sexual or Romantic Interactions or Relationships)**

Counselor–client nonprofessional relationships with clients, former clients, their romantic partners, or their family members should be avoided, except when the interaction is potentially beneficial to the client. (*See A.5.d.*)

§ A.5.d. **Potentially Beneficial Interactions**

When a counselor–client nonprofessional interaction with a client or former client may be potentially beneficial to the client or former client, the counselor must document in case records, prior to the interaction (when feasible), the rationale for such an interaction, the potential benefit, and anticipated consequences for the client or former client and other individuals significantly involved with the client or former client. Such interactions should be initiated with appropriate client consent. Where unintentional harm occurs to the client or former client, or to an individual significantly involved with the client or former client, due to the nonprofessional interaction, the counselor must show evidence of an attempt to remedy such harm. Examples of potentially beneficial interactions include, but are not limited to, attending a formal ceremony (e.g., a wedding/commitment ceremony or graduation); purchasing a service or product provided by a client or former client (excepting unrestricted bartering); hospital visits to an ill family member; mutual membership in a professional association, organization, or community. (*See A.5.c.*)

§ F.3.a. **Relationship Boundaries With Supervisees**

Counseling supervisors clearly define and maintain ethical professional, personal, and social relationships with their supervisees. Counseling supervisors avoid nonprofessional relationships with current supervisees. If supervisors must assume other professional roles (e.g., clinical and administrative supervisor, instructor) with supervisees, they work to minimize potential conflicts and explain to supervisees the expectations and responsibilities associated with each role. They do not engage in any form of nonprofessional interaction that may compromise the supervisory relationship.

TABLE 1: Dual Relationship Ethics *(Continued)*

§ F.10.d. Nonprofessional Relationships

Counselor educations avoid nonprofessional or ongoing professional relationships with students in which there is a risk of potential harm to the student or that may compromise the training experience or grades assigned. In addition, counselor educators do not accept any form of professional services, fees, commissions, reimbursement, or remuneration from a site for student or supervisee placement.

American Association of Pastoral Counselors (AAPC)

§ III.E We recognize the trust placed in and unique power of the therapeutic relationship. While acknowledging the complexity of some pastoral relationships, we avoid exploiting the trust and dependency of clients. We avoid those dual relationships with clients (e.g., business or close personal relationships) which could impair our professional judgement, compromise the integrity of the treatment, and/or use the relationship for our own gain.

§ V.A We do not engage in ongoing counseling relationships with current supervisees, students, and employees.

Note: From the *Ethical Principles of Psychologists and Code of Conduct* by the American Psychological Association. Copyright © 2002 by the American Psychological Association. Reprinted with permission.

The *Code of Ethics* by the American Association for Marriage and Family Therapy is reprinted with permission. Copyright © 2001 by the American Association for Marriage and Family Therapy.

Reprinted from the 2005 ACA *Code of Ethics* by the American Counseling Association. Reprinted with permission. No further reproduction authorized without written permission from the American Counseling Association.

The *Code of Ethics* by the American Association of Pastoral Counselors is reprinted with permission. Copyright © 1994 by the American Association of Pastoral Counselors.

TABLE 2: Reported Disciplinary Actions for Psychologists

August 1983 – April 2003

Compiled from actions reported to the ASPPB Disciplinary Data
System by ASPPB member boards

Reason for Disciplinary Action	Number Disciplined
Sexual/dual relationship with patient	794
Unprofessional/unethical/negligent practice	755
Conviction of crimes	230
Fraudulent acts	172
Improper/inadequate recordkeeping	122
Breach of confidentiality	118
Inadequate or improper supervision	104
Impairment	99
Failure to comply with continuing education requirements	78
Fraud in application for license	50
Other*	451
TOTAL	2,973

*   Some jurisdictions do not report reasons or the reason reported does not
    fall into one of the above listed categories.

    Data from the Association of State and Provincial Psychology Boards
    (ASPPB).

TABLE 3a: California Board of Psychology Disciplinary Data

	92/94	94/95	95/96	96/97	98/99	99/00	00/01	01/02	02/03	03/04	04/05
1. Gross Negligence/Incompetence	27*	27	37	14	8	16	4	6	7	12	0
2. Improper Supervision	0	4	6	14	1	0	0	0	0	0	0
3. Repeat Negligent Acts	-	-	-	-	1	1	1	1	1	2	0
4. Violation of Drug Laws	0	0	0	0	-	-	-	-	-	-	-
5. Self-Abuse of Drugs or Alcohol	0	0	0	0	0	0	1	1	1	1	0
6. Dishonesty/Fraud	3	0	0	3	1	3	1	1	0	2	0
7. Mental Illness	3	2	9	0	3	1	1	0	2	1	0
8. Aiding Unlicensed Practice	0	0	0	0	0	0	0	0	1	0	0
9. General Unprofessional Conduct	3	6	9	11	0	1	2	4	1	2	0
10. Probation Violation	5	2	3	8	3	1	0	1	0	0	0
11. Sexual Misconduct	32	39	16	22	3	2	4	5	2	2	1
12. Conviction of a Crime	11	14	6	32	5	5	5	2	5	2	0
13. Discipline by Another State Board	5	2	6	0	1	3	2	0	2	1	0
14. Voluntary Surrender	0	0	0	0	-	-	-	-	-	-	-
15. Interpersonal Violation	5	0	0	0	0	0	0	0	0	-	-
16. Other	5	2	3	3	0	0	0	0	0	1	0

* Figures appear as percentages. Data from State of California Board of Psychology.

TABLE 3b: Board of Behavioral Sciences Data

Decisions	93/94	94/95	95/96	98/99	99/00	00/01	01/02	02/03	03/04	04/05
				State of California Disciplinary Data						
Fraud	10*	0	3	3	2	2	1	1	0	0
Health & Safety	2	0	0	0	0	0	0	0	0	0
Non-Jurisdictional	0	0	0	N/A	N/A	N/A	-	-	-	-
Competence/Negligence	4	11	16	5	2	4	1	2	9	1
Other	23	0	2	N/A	N/A	N/A	0	0	0	0
Personal Conduct	14	7	18	7	12	8	7	7	3	1
Unprofessional Conduct	46	82	54	4	8	8	8	4	4	2
Unlicensed Activity	2	0	7	1	0	0	0	0	0	0
Sexual Misconduct	-	-	-	14	16	12	13	5	5	1

* Figures are presented as percentages. Covers marriage, family, and child therapists, social workers, and licensed educational psychologists. Data from State of California Board of Behavioral Sciences.

TABLE 4: Social Work Data

Alcohol and Other Substance Abuse 12

Incompetence/Malpractice/Negligence 52

Narcotics Violations 3

Felony 12

Fraud 27

Unprofessional Conduct (including sex) 282

Mental Disorder 3

Allowing Unlicensed Person to Practice 2

Disciplinary Action in Another State 3

Other Reason (Not Classified) 39

Data from the American Association of State Social Work Boards.

Chapter 1

MULTIPLE RELATIONSHIPS AND THEIR CONSEQUENCES FOR MENTAL HEALTH PROFESSIONALS

Dual relationships present unique ethical issues for mental health professionals. Licensing boards, ethics committees, and professional organizations have had difficulty fashioning specific rules regarding dual relationships. The term itself has been a focus of discussion among ethics writers. The premise is that if a mental health professional becomes involved in a secondary relationship, it may be unethical. However, it has been clear from the beginning of this discussion that not all dual relationships are unethical. It has also become clear that a mental health professional could easily be involved in more than two relationships with someone receiving mental health services. Consequently, the term "multiple relationships" replaced dual relationships and is the proper term in vogue today. The rules regarding multiple relationships are evolving. Behnke (2004) explained that although the most recent update of the APA code (2002) has different language, ultimately reasonableness of behavior is of utmost importance ethically.

Nothing written to date concerning multiple relationships has taken a detailed conservative approach that also provides various analytical models to assist one in dealing with ethical issues of this nature. The advice in some of these papers, if followed, may even lead readers into difficulties with their respective licensing boards as well as ethics committees and perhaps even civil liability lawsuits. This book is written to give the reader a conservative model to use in determining which multiple relationships are unethical or illegal and which are acceptable in the field of mental health professionals. Because actual case studies are difficult to find, previous authors have relied on hypothetical circumstances.

Although hypothetical situations are interesting, they are not reality, and their consequences can never actually be known. Of all the cases discussed in this book, there is only one circumstance where a licensing board changed its determination after the professional was involved in the case for several years. As a mental health professional, being charged with an ethical offense is a serious matter. It is one of the most anxiety-provoking experiences a mental health professional can experience, causing an extreme degree of stress to the point that it occupies one's thinking virtually every waking minute and completely alters one's life. Professionals facing an accusation are often very ethical, dedicated, and people of goodwill. A charge investigation can last 5 or more years and cost hundreds of thousands of dollars to the accused in terms of monetary damages or fines; loss or restriction of one's license; probation with various bellicose-sounding conditions, such as having a practice monitor, a paid supervisor, and required mandatory therapy, undergoing a mandatory psychological examination, and meeting with a probation officer every 3 months; having the professional's name published in a state publication; being subject to interviews by licensing board members; loss of insurance coverage; removal from managed care panels; expulsion from hospital privileges; and much more.

The most important consequence of an unlawful or unethical dual relationship is serious and multifaceted harm to a client. Some clients may be so harmed that they lose all belief and trust that psychotherapeutic services may assist them in alleviating disorders from which they suffer. In effect, they seek therapy for one problem and ultimately leave with two problems resulting in a refusal to seek resolution of these problems from the best system available to help the patient. Hope eventually gives way to suspicion and distrust.

Numerous ethical issues present problems for professionals. These include confidentiality, competence, public statements, psychological testing, dealing with other professionals, sexual misconduct, research, psychotherapy practice, financial matters with clients, dealing with supervisors and supervisees, and avoiding harm. Issues of confidentiality are generally easy in that there is one prime directive: **Do Not Disclose**. The rule is easy, and the rationale is very clear and understandable. As Supreme Court Justice Stevens noted in *Jaffee v. Redmond* (1996):

> Treatment by a physician for physical ailments can often proceed successfully on the basis of a physical examination, objective information supplied by the patient, and the results of diagnostic tests. Effective psychotherapy, by contrast, depends upon an atmosphere of confidence and trust in which the patient is willing to make a frank and complete disclosure of facts, emotions, memories and fears. Because of the sensitive nature of the problems for which the individuals consult psychotherapists, disclosure of confidential

communications made during counseling sessions may cause embarrassment or disgrace. For this reason the mere possibility of disclosure may impede development of the confidential relationships necessary for successful treatment. (p. 1928)

After learning the prime directive for confidentiality, therapists then learn the exceptions to the rule. These exceptions fall into two categories: mandatory and permissible. Mandatory exceptions apply to reports of child abuse, elder abuse, dependent adult abuse, violence, dangerous patients, and in some states, therapist abuse. Permissible exceptions apply when the patient is suicidal, when a court-appointed relationship is established, and when a breach of duty in the professional's relationship is alleged or the patient is involved in litigation and claiming emotional or psychological damages. This is one reason that every state in America has rules regarding psychotherapist-patient privilege. (Concerning mental health discipline, only one state – Pennsylvania, in its rules for social workers – has an express prohibition against dual relationships.) Most mental health professionals understand rules of confidentiality and privilege, including both mandatory and permissible exceptions.

As previously mentioned, not all multiple relationships are un-ethical. Factors to be considered in determining which relationships are ethical and which are not include analytical determinations such as conflict of interest, exploitation, loss of objectivity, harm to a patient, or contamination of the relationship itself. This last factor is especially important in that all therapeutic techniques rely on use of the relationship between the therapist and client in order for the client to improve and make necessary changes in his or her life. Of the many psychotherapeutic techniques used by therapists, the primary tool is the relationship itself. An analogy could be made to the surgeon who uses a scalpel to perform surgery in order to treat the disease of the patient. Use of a dirty or contaminated scalpel may harm the patient or even be lethal by infecting the patient. Consequently, if the thera-peutic relationship becomes infected, the patient may be damaged for life, and that patient will eventually infect others.

There is an additional aspect of multiple relationships that has changed over the years. In the past, rules and prohibitions about mul-tiple relationships applied only to psychotherapy relationships, thereby causing the analysis of patients to be much easier during that period. The first or primary relationship always began with a determination of whether a psychotherapist-patient relationship existed. That constituted relationship number one. An illustration makes this point more clear:

Psychotherapist-Patient Relationship? Yes = Relationship #1

Once the primary relationship was determined, it was critical to determine if other relationships existed. Examples of other relationships could be a sexual partner, friend, colleague, business partner, neighbor, relative, prior sexual partner, lender, or borrower, to name a few. The illustration could be mapped out to ascertain whether there is a second relationship as follows:

Psychotherapist-Patient = Relationship #1
Neighbor-Neighbor = Relationship #2
Aunt-Cousin = Relationship #3

In the example presented above, it is clear there are three different relationships which will automatically raise the issue of a role relationship problem. The ethical and legal issue always begins and ends with a determination of whether there is a psychotherapist-patient relationship. In recent times, multiple relationship ethics have been applied for other types of mental health relationships, which has greatly expanded the circumstances where unethical conduct may exist, even in an unsuspecting professional. Some current examples of these expanded relationships that may trigger the multiple relationship issue and force a psychologist or social worker to conduct a more in-depth analysis include:

Supervisor–Supervisee
Teacher–Student
Forensic Service Provider–Object of Services
Consultant–Consultee
Worker's Compensation Evaluator–Evaluee

Once a professional relationship has been established, it is incumbent on the mental health provider to ascertain whether there are any other relationships. Heretofore, the primary focus in published papers concerning multiple relationships was in dealing with psychotherapy patients. As we have seen, many other possibilities for multiple relationships exist, most of which have not been previously discussed in depth but are covered in this book. In addition, this book examines the problem of inadvertent multiple relationships which often arise in rural communities.

One of the most recent edited books written on multiple relationships argues that many multiple relationships are helpful and that rules prohibiting them are arcane and should be eliminated (Lazarus & Zur, 2002). Although the aforementioned book is an important work on the subject, there is a strong likelihood that, if a professional follows the advice of the authors, that professional is likely to become the object of a disciplinary action. Unfortunately, in 2006, we live in a world where mental health professionals face scrutiny of their work at a level never seen before at any point in professional practice. Presently, there are now six primary ways professionals can face negative consequences for their actions. First, licensing boards have been created to protect the public and regulate mental health professions, including social workers, psychologists, psychiatrists, marriage and family therapists, licensed professional counselors, licensed educational counselors, psychiatric nurse practitioners, and psychiatric technicians. In the state of California, the Board of Psychology receives approximately 600 complaints against licensees each year. Regulatory boards have the power both to license professionals and to discipline them, including revocation of a license for egregious offenses, many of which involve multiple relationships. As previously mentioned, a regulatory investigation can last for many years, draining a professional emotionally, financially, and professionally.

Second, many statutes governing mental health practice have criminal law implications. If violated, a mental health professional who engages in any form of multiple relationship may face loss of liberty, along with other consequences. There was a California case in which a psychiatrist engaged in sexual contact with a patient in his office and billed for services rendered under an insurance program for the indigent in the state of California known as Medi-Cal. The outcome of this case resulted in this psychiatrist losing his license and also being sent to prison.

Third, violation of prohibitions against multiple relationships may lead to the filing of a lawsuit against the professional for monetary damages. Patients are becoming savvier regarding how to use civil litigation against their mental health practitioners, including evaluators. In *Pettus v. Cole* (1996), an individual sued two evaluators who were hired by an employer to determine whether the plaintiff was able to perform the functions and duties of his work. Although the trial court dismissed the case, the California Appellate Court of the Third District found merit in the claim. There were dual relationships in the *Pettus* case, although the civil suit was based on another ethical matter. So, in essence, not only can professionals face loss of their license, as well as loss of their liberty, but they may face a lawsuit for a multiple relationship violation.

Fourth, an ethics complaint can be filed with the state or national ethics committee of the professional organization of which the provider is a member. The harshest punishment resulting from an ethics action is the member's expulsion from the organization. However, disciplinary action from national ethics committees are published and generally sent to licensing boards, which, in turn, trigger a licensing case. In addition, expulsion from an organization for unethical conduct can lead to many other punitive results such as loss of hospital privileges. In some cases an angry client may pursue all possible avenues of adverse action against the professional.

Fifth, angry and upset consumers of mental health services may file a complaint against the professional at his or her workplace. City, county, state, and federal governmental agencies, courts, and private employers generally have procedures to handle complaints from the public. A serious complaint could result in termination of employment or negative information being placed in the personnel file of the professional.

Finally, clients may complain to managed health care entities. Most insurance carriers and managed health care entities have public relations departments designed to handle complaints against a provider. Complaints filed in this setting are often handled swiftly. The most serious result is removal from the panel of experts used by the company. If the provider does a substantial amount of business with the company, expulsion could lead to considerable loss of income. Further, some states, such as California, require that a report be made to the licensing board of the provider where any adverse action may be taken against that individual.

In summary, the six common methods in which a professional can face negative consequences for his or her actions and which would aversely affect his or her practice are:

1. Licensing board complaint
2. Criminal complaint
3. Civil litigation
4. Ethics complaint to professional organizations
5. Complaint to one's employer
6. Insurance or managed care company complaint

Chapter 2

ANALYSIS OF MULTIPLE RELATIONSHIP ISSUES

The therapist should ask a series of questions before determining whether a therapeutic or other professional relationship could be harmful or exploitative and/or if it will interfere with the professional's therapy. This will provide the therapist with a formula for analyzing whether a conflict of interest may exist based upon the relationship the professional has established with the client. The therapist should ask the following questions:

1. *Is there a professional relationship* or *are you providing psychological services to the person?*

   Examples:

Therapy	Testing/evaluation
Consultation	Evaluation
Supervision	Psychological teaching
Trial consultation	Forensic professional
Managed care analyst/evaluator	
Corporate manager/executive	
Licensing or ethics board member	

2. *Is there more than one relationship with the person?*
3. *What are the relationships? (List them)*

   Examples:

Patient-Therapist	Lover-Lover

4. *Are the secondary relationships in the prohibited class?* The "prohibited class" of relationships refers to a number of multiple

relationships that experience has taught us are likely to be harmful, lead to exploitation, and create confusion or contamination in the primary relationship. Mental health professions should avoid these types of multiple relationships.

Examples:

Former sexual partners	Business associates
Coworkers	Family members
Spouses	Friends
Relatives	Students
Teachers	Current sexual partners
Employees	

5. *If not in the prohibited class, is the secondary relationship likely to create a conflict of interest and/or cause harm to the patient?*

Examples:

Cause harm: actual or possible
Reduce the effectiveness of the service
Lead to a loss of objectivity
Exploit the client
Role confusion
Restrict the patient's actions
Restrict the therapist's actions
Prevent the patient from continuing therapy
Lead to a legal dispute
Cause the patient to be upset by the secondary relationship

6. *How easy is it to avoid the secondary relationship/conflict of interest?* For example, secondary relationships may be more difficult to avoid in rural areas where there are fewer providers of all services.

7. *Has an independent and objective consultant approved of the secondary relationship or proposed conduct?* It is recommended that therapists obtain the assistance from a consultant such as a senior clinician, attorney, or ethics committee member. The consultant should not be a friend. The consultant should be someone who is objective and professionally knowledgeable. Selection of a nonobjective consultant could lead to faulty reasoning and bad decision making. (See Appendices B and C [pp. 169-174] for guidelines on choosing a qualified consultant.)

8. *How will the relationship or conduct reflect upon the profession?* The flow chart in Figure 1 (pp. 28-30) can be used to guide the professional to act appropriately.

The categories noted in the part of Figure 1 labeled "Analysis of Potential Harm" (p. 30) are defined below.

Explanation of Flow Chart

Environment

This refers to the place where the secondary relationship occurs— outside of the professional environment or within it. This is quite important. If the contact occurs outside of the therapist's office or in a more private environment, one would expect more conflict for the client, generally. Having lunch with a client in a crowded and open restaurant is different from having dinner in a quiet, romantic restaurant. Of course, there are many cases of therapists acting out sexually in their offices with clients. This factor is not in any way dispositive.

Purpose/Motive of the Activity

The therapist's motivation is important to examine, assuming that there is an objective analysis of such a motive. Is the motivation of the therapist's conduct established to satisfy a therapist's nonprofessional need, or is it designed to promote the client's best interest? Is the conduct solely or primarily designed to satisfy a well-documented therapeutic objective or goal that is identified in the client's treatment plan? If the conduct is in the interest of the client, it may be acceptable, provided, however, that the determination of what is in the best interest of the client is made objectively.

The Extent of Contact

This factor involves the extent of physical contact with the client. Does the contact involve a brief handshake or sexual intercourse? One is more cursory and accepted, while the other is intimate and extensive. The greater and more intimate the physical contact, the more likely it will be harmful. Sexual behaviors involving activities such as intercourse, oral sexual contact, sexually oriented massages, long embraces, or long kisses which are lip to lip and involve lengthy intimate contact are known to cause harm to the client and the therapeutic relationship. Other behavior, such as a short hug offered at the appropriate time, such as at the end of a difficult therapeutic session and with no sexual connotation, may be helpful to the client and the relationship between the therapist and client.

Methodology Used by the Therapist

Does the therapist use coercion, force, or actual or perceived threats to obtain a client's acquiescence to the questionable conduct? Over a period of time, has the therapist engaged in behavior designed to magnify the power differential with the client? Does the therapist in any way threaten the client, thereby forcing the client into the proposed conduct? Threats by the therapist could take the form of reports to child protective service agencies, employers, police, relatives, or others who may be able to use confidential information about a client adversely. Does the therapist agree to reduce the client's bill in exchange for the client's involvement in the secondary relationship?

Tendency of the Behavior to Create Confusion

Does the behavior or secondary relationship create confusion for the client regarding the therapeutic purpose of the primary relationship? Will the client have difficulties because of the confusion?

Appearance

This refers to the appearance of the activity with the client. If the behavior of the therapist appears to others to be against the best interest of the client, or harmful, it should be prohibited. If others who may be considering seeking treatment by the therapist may be disinclined to do so because they observe the behavior in question, the mental health professional might consider refraining from the intended conduct.

Context

This calls for an analysis of the context in which the conduct of the therapist occurred. Did the conduct occur in the context of a planned or structured therapeutic activity established to be in the interest of the client, such as in a therapeutic group recreational visit to a bowling alley, as an example, or was it more likely to be harmful to the client, such as an intimate dinner with no therapeutic purpose intended?

Prohibition of Future Therapy

If the conduct in question would have an effect on the client's choice to pursue therapy with the therapist in the future, it is likely to be both harmful to the client and a conflict of interest. When therapeutic boundaries are maintained such that a client could easily come back for treatment at a later time, it is clearly in the client's interest to preserve such an option.

Objectivity

This calls for a determination as to whether the objectivity of the therapist, as well as the client, will be diminished by the activity in question. Behavior such as a therapist having a sexual relationship with a client clearly impairs the objectivity of both the therapist and the client. Impairment of objectivity must certainly be harmful to the client.

Free Will

This refers to the extent to which the free will of a client is impaired by the conduct in question. If the conduct in question is not aimed at the best interest of the client, it may be harmful if the client's will is impeded. Arguably, the development of positive feelings by the client toward the therapist may adversely affect free will. However, if the conduct is still aimed at the best interest of the client, it may be helpful. The therapist should always seek consultation to help ascertain what is in the best interest of the client.

Strength of the Client

Rarely has this factor been considered in an analysis of the harm to the client. The client who is mentally healthy is clearly in a better position to make an independent decision about the secondary relationship. A client in a psychiatric hospital or one with a borderline personality disorder is not a client who should be involved in any type of dual relationship with a mental health professional.

The final portion of the analysis must focus upon the mental health of the professional. There is no justification for engaging in conduct or conflicts of interest, as well as multiple relationships, which fall in the prohibited class. Many mental health professionals engage in boundary violations when they are vulnerable, depressed, or when they are experiencing significant psychosocial stressors. However, for those areas less clear, the mental health of the professional should factor into the equation. That is, the more mentally healthy the professional, the more latitude should be given for involvement in multiple relationships that are not necessarily harmful. The less mentally healthy the professional, the less that person should stray from strict professional boundaries. Those who have certain types of personality disorders themselves may be more likely to engage in boundary violations. Depressed, vulnerable, personality disordered, and stressed therapists should receive less latitude than those who are not impaired. Again, the latitude applies only to those situations where the conduct in question is not in the prohibited class and may not be harmful or exploitative to the client. Some case examples will illustrate the use of the model.

Case Examples*

Case #1

A social worker is treating a 12-year-old patient for anger she experiences in school. The adolescent has a mild adjustment disorder diagnosis and possible ADHD. The adolescent and the psychologist live in a small town in Idaho with a population of 15,000. The psychologist keeps no confidential material at his home. He is mentally healthy and has kept very tight boundaries in the past. Given the managed care insurance plan for the patient, as well as the nature of her problems, the psychologist anticipates that she will only need six sessions of supportive therapy.

The psychologist is divorced and has a 3-year-old daughter. He has joint custody. One of the stresses for the patient is a lack of money, although she tries to babysit every weekend. The psychologist learns during the fourth session that his wife knows the patient incidentally. The patient becomes aware that the psychologist and his wife must be at a very important meeting on a Friday evening. She offers to babysit for her regular fee of $6.00 per hour. Now we will examine this situation in light of the model.

There is a professional relationship. There are multiple relationships (therapist-patient; parent-babysitter). The secondary relationship is not in the prohibited class. Using the harm analysis, there is some concern raised because the secondary relationship will take place in the home of the psychologist. However, there is no confidential material there. The purpose of the activity will meet the needs of both the patient and the therapist. The activity is not clearly directed at promoting the best interests of the client exclusively. There will be limited contact, none of which will be physical. The therapist is using a short-term treatment model making it less likely for a powerful attachment to occur between the patient and himself. The behavior may create some minor confusion, although the role of a babysitter is not completely opposite of a therapeutic relationship. There is no evidence that objectivity of the therapist may be adversely affected nor will the free will of the client be injured in any way. Both the therapist and the patient are relatively healthy. Using the model there are many negatives that might make the activity unwise and probably would be determined to be unethical by most licensing boards as well as professional associations despite the fact that the specific ethical principles and standards may not make the dual relationship completely unethical. When in doubt, be conservative and do not engage in this type of conduct.

---

* Names and characteristics in all case examples have been changed to protect privacy.

Change some of the facts in this scenario and there would be a different result. Make the environment urban, the patient seriously ill, the psychologist a sexual predator, and the therapy analytic, and these changes would lead to the conclusion that the activity would create a conflict of interest.

Case #2

A social worker, who is psychologically healthy, is treating a 7-year-old female who is in a residential treatment center. The 7-year-old was physically abused by both her mother and father resulting in her removal from the home and termination of their parental rights. The social worker provides weekly treatment and the patient responds. The patient has a variety of symptoms, including depression, anxiety, social withdrawal, poor school performance, difficulty concentrating, memory problems, and uncontrollable crying at times. She has no independent source of money, and the residential treatment facility has a limited budget. The social worker takes the girl to the local town one day and purchases several appropriate outfits for the child. In addition, the social worker invited the child to her home for Thanksgiving dinner. An independent consultant concluded that the behavior is appropriate.

Using the model, it is clear that a professional relationship exists. There is also a secondary relationship. The secondary relationship is not in the prohibited class. The behavior in question is in the best interests of the client. It is unlikely there would be an adverse effect on future therapy because the therapeutic boundary in the primary relationship is not contaminated. Likewise, there does not appear to be any adverse effect on objectivity. The appearance of the conduct would not discredit the profession in any way. Finally, the objective consultant concludes the conduct is appropriate. Given this scenario, the relationship would be considered ethical.

Case #3

A 28-year-old psychologist is working in a county inpatient psychiatric center. She is treating a 16-year-old male patient who has been psychotic and who has an IQ of 85. She uses a long-term dynamic treatment method with the patient. She expresses her attraction for the patient in a session. Later she hugs him after each of her sessions. She continually asks him if he is attracted to her. After one session she gives him $100 as spending money. He is surprised and elated. He asks what he can do to pay her back. She looks seductively into his eyes and tells him she will think of something. The psychologist herself has been treated for a borderline personality disorder and discontinued treatment after a verbal altercation with her therapist.

In this scenario there is a professional relationship and there is a secondary relationship. The secondary relationship is not yet in the prohibited class. The patient and therapist both are psychologically impaired to the extent that the psychologist should not involve herself in any unusual secondary role relationship. The conduct in question is likely to create role confusion because there are clear personal sexual overtones alluded to during therapy, and the cash is an unusual gift to a patient who does not need the gift. The motive of the activity is suspect and is not likely to be in the best interest of the patient. Further, the objectivity of the psychologist and the patient are likely to be impaired in this instance. The psychologist is using a long-term treatment model which depends on the purity of the relationship over a period of time. The conduct may ultimately impede progress in the future or lead the patient to want to discontinue treatment with the psychologist. The appearance brings discredit upon the profession. In this case, a consultant was never contacted. Clearly there is a major conflict of interest in the actions of the psychologist. The analysis in this case would lead to an unequivocal conclusion that the behavior is unethical and should be avoided.

Case #4

A 54-year-old patient has been in cognitive-behavioral therapy with a supportive therapy overtone for the past year and a half. She has decided to terminate therapy with the approval of the psychologist. After the last session the psychologist and the patient go to lunch in a very public setting as a celebration of the success of treatment.

This case involves a clear professional relationship with a secondary relationship that involves going to lunch with the patient. However, the conduct is not in the prohibited class. The context is one involving a time-limited contact to symbolize success in therapy. Consequently, there does not appear to be an extratherapeutic reason for the conduct. Objectivity is unimpaired in both the patient and the psychologist, and both are relatively healthy at this point. Likewise, there does not appear to be an adverse effect on the free will of either the patient or the psychologist. In addition, the patient will most likely not be uncomfortable about pursuing future therapy with the psychologist as the result of going to lunch with him. It is unlikely that the lunch will create any confusion in the primary relationship. Under the model the conduct would be considered ethical.

Case #5

A 29-year-old psychological assistant of a psychologist needs to obtain therapy to complete a graduate school requirement. He does not have any money to pay for therapy. He approaches his psychologist supervisor who agrees to provide therapy.

In this case there is a primary professional relationship. There is also a secondary relationship. Further, the secondary relationship is in the prohibited class. Hence, according to the model, the psychological assistant must be referred elsewhere for therapy.

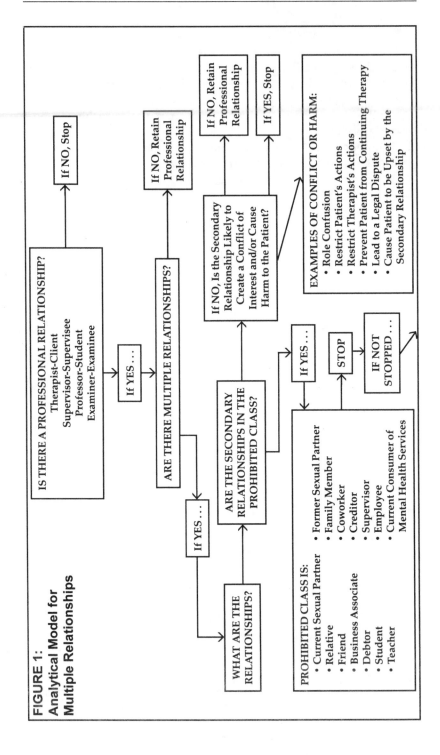

FIGURE 1:
Analytical Model for
Multiple Relationships

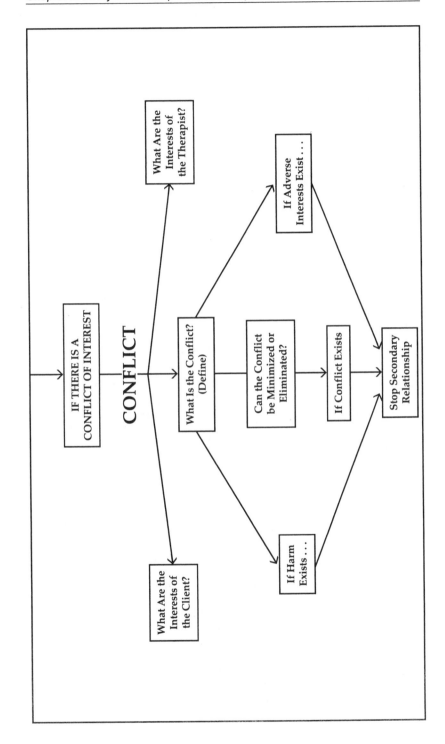

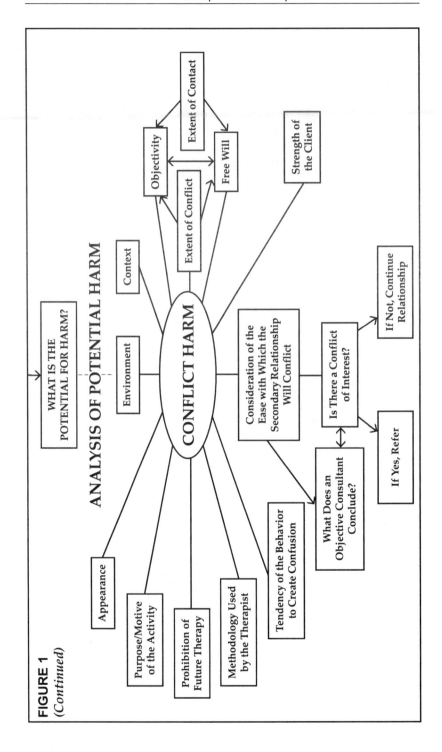

FIGURE 1
(Continued)

Chapter 3

DETERMINING WHICH MULTIPLE
RELATIONSHIPS ARE A PROBLEM*

The primary problem is determining which multiple relationships are unethical or illegal and which behaviors create a conflict of interest for the mental health professional. There are several theoretical positions that are helpful in conducting an analysis of the therapist's behavior or multiple relationship. First, there are the "boundary theorists," who conclude that there should be a very strict and virtually impenetrable boundary between a therapist and client (Gabbard, 1989; Gabbard & Lester, 1995; Gutheil & Gabbard, 1993; Hatcher, 1993; Pope & Vasquez, 2001). Many boundary theorists believe that any behavior that crosses the therapeutic boundary is unethical and should be prohibited. The therapist's role is to maintain strict therapeutic boundaries, which should be acted upon based upon a therapeutic motive with methods that are recognized to be within the role of a therapist treating a client. Any other conduct is prohibited and considered inappropriate. Consequently, in order to establish and maintain a professional relationship between the therapist and client, all contact and interactions between the two are to be in a therapeutic setting. Crossing the therapeutic boundary by entering into a nontherapeutic relationship is considered unethical.

A second position is that of the "harm theorists." These theorists rely on ethics code principles that preclude professionals from engaging in behavior that is harmful to clients. They rely on ethics code provisions such as APA Standards 3.04, AAMFT Principle 1.3, NASW Principle 1.06, and American Psychiatric Association Section

---

* Portions of this chapter from *Dual Relationships and Psychotherapy*, A. Lazarus and O. Zur. Copyright © 2002 by Springer Publishing, Inc., New York, NY 10036. Used with permission.

1(1). The relevant APA Standard (3.04) is referred to as Avoiding Harm and states: "Psychologists take reasonable steps to avoid harming their clients/patients, students, supervisees, research participants, organizational clients, and others with whom they work, and to minimize harm where it is foreseeable and unavoidable." Behavior that is harmful to the client is unethical. Any relationship that causes harm that is foreseeable by the therapist is also considered unethical. Any analysis of the propriety or impropriety of a relationship is focused upon the harm that is likely to occur as the result of that relationship.

A third theoretical orientation is the fiduciary duty theory. A fiduciary duty is a concept from law that is the highest form of obligation owed to one person by another. A fiduciary is "a person having a legal duty, created by his undertaking, to act primarily for the benefit of another in matters connected with his undertaking" (Gifis, 1984, p. 185). This concept is also mentioned in one of the latest books dealing with interpretation of the new APA code of ethics (Knapp & Vandecreek, 2003).

The fiduciary in mental health practice owes a solemn clinical, not necessarily financial, duty to the client. The professional must watch out for the best interest of the client and engage in behavior that is in keeping with the therapeutic interests of the client. The fiduciary theory creates broad duties and responsibilities for the therapist, not only to prevent harm to the client, but also to work toward the most positive and helpful conduct in support of the client. The therapist must be a watchdog of the client and serve as a protector and preserver of the client's psychological assets and to assist in their growth, just as a trust administrator is responsible for a client's financial assets. In law, a trust fund administrator can be removed and sued for failing to maintain trust fund growth at a reasonable level commensurate with current economic circumstances.

Ebert (1997) created a fourth theoretical orientation that is called constitutional conduct. In this model the therapist is required to act in the best constitutional interests of the client. However, ethics code provisions are also required to be constructed with the constitutional rights of mental health professionals in mind, as well as those of the clients. The model is based upon the recognition of universal ethical principles and the existence of fundamental rights. The duty to adhere to these principles comes from a deep commitment to do the right thing, not solely by working for the client in an effort to avoid punishment or to prevent harm to a patient, but based upon the dedication to conduct oneself with virtue in accordance with these universal principles.

The best and most practical approach for professionals to take is to adopt a model that considers all of the theoretical positions. Hence, a mental health professional should act in constitutionally appropriate ways with his or her clients as well as assume there are fiduciary duties owed to the client, and always act in a manner to preclude harm to a client. They should consider the Universal Declaration of Human Rights (United Nations, 1948). A method of doing all of the above is to consider maintaining relatively strict therapeutic boundaries.

Another practical method of avoiding conflict and multiple relationships that are exploitative in nature is to use the analytical model presented in Chapter 2 and apply it to circumstances where the ethics of any proposed conduct are in question.

A final factor to be considered in the analysis is the psychological state of the professional. Professionals with personality disorders, or even strong personality traits such as narcissism, borderline, or histrionics, should refrain from voluntarily entering into multiple relationships and should be ever watchful of conflict situations. Professionals who are experiencing an adjustment disorder should be extra careful, while those who are psychotic or severely depressed should never have professional contact with consumers until they are more stable. There may, however, be more latitude in the more ambiguous areas of contact for those who are psychologically healthy, strong, and have unyielding impulse control.

By tracing the decisions and comments by the APA over the past 10 years and examining the thinking of experts in ethics who have published, we know the following dual relationships are unethical:

1. *Sexual contact with a patient is unethical.*

   On this point there is consistent thinking. APA Standard 10.05 (APA, 2002) expressly prohibits such conduct (see also Haas & Malouf, 2005; Koocher & Keith-Spiegel, 1998; Pope & Vasquez, 1991, 2001). All state licensing boards agree on the ethics standards regarding this issue. Also, in some states, a new trend is taking place determining and establishing that sexual conduct with a patient is a criminal offense. An example of such a state is California, where the California Business and Professions Code, Section 729, criminalizes such activity. (Also see every major mental health organization's code of ethics.)

2. *Treatment of close friends, family members, and/or employees is unethical.*

   (See APA Standard 3.05 [APA, 2002].)

3. *Treatment of students is unethical, generally.*

(APA, 2002, Standard 7.05; AAMFT, 2001, Section 4.2.) Treatment of a student in which there is close contact or involvement as a faculty member in the supervision or evaluation of the student is considered unethical by the APA Committee on Professional Standards (1987) and by many writers. However, the 1987 committee report obfuscated the problem by offering an analytical framework to be applied to professor-therapist situations. There seems to be a difference in the type of student relationship which will determine whether the dual relationship that develops is unethical. This has been given more attention recently.

4. *Bartering, whereby services are exchanged for other services, may be unethical.*

(However see APA, 2002, Standard 6.05, allowing barter in some circumstances.)

5. *Entering into a business relationship with a patient is unethical.*

6. *Entering into a business relationship with an ex-patient is often considered to be unethical.*

7. *A minister/pastor who is also a psychologist who provides counseling to a church member will likely be judged to have engaged in unethical conduct.*

(APA Committee on Professional Standards, 1987.) Does this ruling fly squarely in the face of religious practice for several hundred years? Is the psychologist's and patient's freedom of religion suddenly and arbitrarily restricted?

8. *Establishing a Debtor-Creditor relationship with a client/patient by billing or accepting payments is unethical.*

This dual relationship, which is often harmful to the patient and certainly creates the risk of exploitation, has been found to be unethical. It is seldom discussed, because the logic used to prohibit other types of conflictive dual relationships could not support this type of relationship. Consider the relative harm in going to lunch with a patient versus allowing a bill to accrue to $500, thereafter sending a late notice to the patient. When payment has not been made, the bill is sent to collection and the professional/psychologist takes the patient to small claims court. Yet the former (going to lunch) is considered unethical and the latter (letting the bill accrue) is not. The latter is supported by self-serving rationalizations and basic denial of the effect such practices will have on the patient. Current ethics policies would allow clients to make monthly payments to psychologists, a fact which creates a revolving credit plan and generally requires disclosure under the Federal Truth and Lending Act.

Areas Subject to Confusion

1. Socializing with a patient may or may not be unethical, depending upon such factors as the stability of the patient, interests or needs of the therapist, and whether the activity may cause harm or lead to exploitation of the client.
2. Socializing with an ex-patient is not prohibited.
3. Bartering with a patient, whereby goods offered by the patient are given in exchange for psychotherapy, may not be unethical.
4. Sexual contact with an ex-patient may not always be judged to be unethical.
5. Treatment of a former student may be allowed.
6. Developing a friendship with an ex-patient may not always be prohibited.
7. Treatment of an individual employed in a facility where the psychologist works may be ethical and may be unethical.
8. Buying goods from a patient may be unethical.
9. Treatment of a current student may be ethical. This conclusion by the committee (APA Committee on Professional Standards, 1987) has never been overruled, although it is hard to believe this would be considered ethical in 2006. Certainly ethics writers such as Pope and Vasquez (1991, 2001) would never consider this practice acceptable.
10. Performing an evaluation and treatment on the same client may or may not be ethical, depending upon when each is performed.
11. Traveling in the same professional circles as a patient may be unethical.
12. Psychologists who treat other psychologists may not be able to belong to associations or attend professional functions.

13. Psychologists who have consenting sexual relationships with their employees may be unethical.
14. Socializing with students may be unethical.
15. Psychologists who date each other and work in the same setting may be behaving unethically.
16. Exchanging gifts with a patient may be unethical.
17. Charging money for supervision in which the hours will be used for licensure purposes may be unethical.
18. Having a social relationship with a supervisee may be unethical.
19. Hiring a former student or supervisee may be unethical.

I do not believe that all of the preceding are, in fact, unethical. The prior interpretations of dual relationship cases by the APA, as well as the principles promulgated by Pope and others, raise serious questions about which conduct is considered to be ethical and that which is considered to be unethical.

Chapter 4

SEX WITH CLIENTS*

All of the major ethics codes of professional mental health associations prohibit sexual conduct with current patients. A summary of the prohibitions appears in Table 5 (p. 38).

Therapy is a very intimate experience for the therapist and the client. In a typical therapy situation, the therapist sits in an enclosed room with a client discussing the most intimate aspects of the client's life. It is artificial in that the total focus of the conversation during the therapy hour is on the client's private life, including his or her inner feelings, thoughts, impulses, and experiences. Sexual feelings are very common in therapy (Pope, 1994). It is normal for a client to develop positive feelings for the therapist, which often include the development of sexual feelings. This is referred to as transference, although cognitive-behavioral therapists do not necessarily accept the concept of transference. It is clearly agreed upon that sexual contact between a therapist and a client is unethical. The ethical problems associated with sexual intimacies with a person receiving professional services are well documented (Bates & Brodsky, 1989; Gabbard & Lester, 1995; Herlihy & Corey, 1992; Peterson, 1992; Pope, 1994; Pope & Bouhoutsos, 1986). Every professional should have this literature in his or her library.

It is also normal for a therapist to develop positive feelings for the client. This is often referred to as countertransference. These terms are used quite often in licensing and ethics cases, although they are psychodynamic theoretical terms, which do not necessarily have a scientific

---

* Portions of this chapter from *Dual Relationships and Psychotherapy*, A. Lazarus and O. Zur. Copyright © 2002 by Springer Publishing, Inc., New York, NY 10036. Used with permission.

TABLE 5: Sex With Clients

American Psychological Association (APA)

§ 10.05 Sexual Intimacies With Current Therapy Clients/Patients. Psychologists do not engage in sexual intimacies with current clients/patients.

§ 10.07 Therapy With Former Sexual Partners. Psychologists do not accept as therapy clients/patients with whom they have engaged in sexual intimacies.

American Association for Marriage and FamilyTherapy (AAMFT)

§ 1.4 Sexual intimacy with clients is prohibited.

National Association of Social Workers (NASW)

§ 1.09 (a) Social workers should under no circumstances engage in sexual activities or sexual contact with current clients, whether such contact is consensual or forced.

(b) Social workers should not engage in sexual activities or sexual contact with clients' relatives or other individuals with whom clients maintain a close personal relationship when there is a risk of exploitation or potential harm to the client. Sexual activity or sexual contact with clients' relatives or other individuals with whom clients maintain a personal relationship has the potential to be harmful to the client and may make it difficult for the social worker and client to maintain appropriate professional boundaries. Social workers—not their clients, their clients' relatives, or other individuals with whom the client maintains a personal relationship—assume the full burden for setting clear, appropriate, and culturally sensitive boundaries.

American Psychiatric Association

§ 2.1 The necessary intensity of the treatment relationship may tend to activate sexual and other needs and fantasies on the part of both patient and psychiatrist, while weakening the objectivity necessary for control. . . . Sexual activity with a current or former patient is unethical.

American Counseling Association (ACA)

§ A.5.a. **Current Clients**

Sexual or romantic counselor-client interactions or relationships with current clients, their romantic partners, or their family members are prohibited.

American Association of Pastoral Counselors (AAPC)

§ III.G All forms of behavior or harassment with clients are unethical, even when the client invites or consents to such behavior or involvement.

basis established to support the existence of such a phenomenon. In behavioral terms, a client and therapist interact in a mutually reinforcing and positive experience, creating positive feelings for both. Nevertheless, it is universally recognized that because therapy and other psychological services involve intimacy often not experienced regularly by clients, or even by therapists, both therapist and client may become attracted to one other.

The nature of the problem has been well documented in professional literature (Nugent, 1994). It has been determined through research that 7% to 15% of all male therapists have had sexual contact with a client (D. S. Solursh, L. F. Solursh, & Williams, 1993). The most frequent reason for discipline before the California Board of Psychology over the past 10 years involves allegations of sexual misconduct by a psychologist. More than one-half of all adjudicated cases involve sexual behavior between a psychologist and a client. All types of sexual conduct are prohibited, not just sexual intercourse. Sexual conduct includes sexual intercourse, intimate touching of the genitals of the client, oral sex, kissing, any type of sexual hugging, sexual talk designed to appeal to one's prurient interest and not directed to addressing a client's problems, and any other physical contact of a sexual nature between the therapist and the client. Sexual conduct with a current patient is a crime punishable by imprisonment in California (California Business and Professions Code Section 729).

Such misconduct contaminates the relationship between the professional and the client. The key tool used by mental health professionals in practicing their craft is the therapeutic relationship established between the professional and the client. Adding a highly emotional relationship with sexual conduct contaminates the tool of the craft, not unlike a surgeon using a dirty scalpel to operate on a patient. There is absolutely no excuse for engaging in sexual conduct with a patient, supervisee, student, person being evaluated, or any other consumer of mental health services. It is wrong, it is illegal, and it is harmful to clients/patients. In a case in California illustrative of the problem, a female psychologist provided therapy to a female patient, and the relationship developed into an unethical multiple relationship (*In the Matter of the Accusation Against Barbara Grimes*, 1997). The patient was quite psychologically ill and required hospitalization. Apparently the patient was encouraged to go to the home of the psychologist. The psychologist and the patient went shopping together, played tennis, shared meals at the home of the psychologist, and spent the night together. In December of 1990 the psychologist and her fiancé went on a skiing trip with her patient and her patient's husband to Mammoth Mountain in California. In January 1991, the psychologist went on a skiing trip to Utah with the patient and another person. In the same month, the psychologist went to Kauai with the patient and the patient's husband, along with the psychologist's father and his girlfriend. In addition, the patient's husband painted the cabin of the father of the psychologist. At one point the patient owed the psychologist $3,900, which was forgiven by the psychologist. Despite the fact that the patient had been hospitalized approximately six times, the psychologist entered into a sexual relationship with the patient. They had dinner together, shared a hot tub spa together, and drank wine. In addition, the psychologist and the patient spent the night together in the same bed. As a result, this psychologist lost her license and clearly caused severe harm to the patient.

Reasons to Engage in Sexual Conduct With a Client

<u>NONE</u>. There is never a reason to engage in sexual contact with a client.

Reasons Not to Engage in Sexual Conduct With a Client

1. It may be extremely harmful to the client.
2. Many victims of prior sexual abuse become involved in sexual conduct with their therapists. It is a form of revictimization.
3. It is a violation of the professional licensing laws established in the United States and can result in revocation of one's license.
4. It is a violation of the professional ethics codes of mental health professionals and can result in expulsion from a professional association.
5. It may be an indication of impairment on the part of the therapist.
6. Some victims of therapist abuse may engage in sexualized behavior in hopes that a safe therapist will not take advantage of them.
7. It is harmful to the public's perception of the profession of those in mental health and may hinder others from entering into therapy.
8. In several states, it constitutes criminal conduct and can result in a jail sentence.
9. If the client does not have the capacity to consent to the sexual conduct, the conduct will be considered a felony.

When confronted with a situation in which you are attracted to a client, it is important to take the following steps:

1. Perform a self-check to ascertain why you have become attracted to the client.
2. Discuss the case with an objective consultant, someone who will provide you with an honest assessment of the situation. (For guidelines in choosing a competent consultant, see Appendices B & C [pp. 169-174].)
3. Take all steps necessary to ensure that you will not act out your sexual impulses with the client.
4. If you are inclined to act out, then refer your client to another therapist and do not act out, even after the referral has been made. In at least one state, it is a crime to terminate therapy for the purposes of engaging in sexual contact with a client (California Business and Professions Code Section 729).
5. Consider entering into therapy yourself if you have seriously entertained the notion of acting out with your client.
6. Assign yourself to complete a bibliotherapy by reading professional papers on the adverse effects of sexual conduct between a therapist and a client.
7. When aware of sexual fantasies about your client, consider using cognitive-behavioral techniques similar to those used in relapse prevention with sex offenders (Perkens, 1991).
8. Remind yourself that if you are caught, you will be considered a sexual offender.
9. Challenge your own thinking when you begin to rationalize why it would be acceptable for you to engage in sexual contact with a client.
10. Consider reentering supervision or obtaining a practice monitor.
11. Consider taking a break from your practice if you genuinely feel you cannot control yourself.

Rules for Ethical Practice

Rule #1: Do not have sex with your clients—ever!

1. Sexual relationships with clients are prohibited by law and by every ethical code in the mental health profession.
2. The California Business and Professions Code Section 729 makes it a crime to engage in sexual intercourse, sodomy, oral copulation, or any other sexual contact with a patient. The first

time offense would be a misdemeanor, and repeat offenses would constitute a felony. As previously noted, sexual contact does not only need to be intercourse, it can also be in the form of intimate touching of the genitals of the client, oral sex, kissing, and any type of sexual hugging.

3. Sexual contact is expressly prohibited between a therapist and patient under every mental health profession licensing statute. Consider the California Code dealing with licensing:

> Unprofessional conduct shall include . . . any act of sexual abuse, or sexual relations with a patient or former patient within two years following termination of therapy, or sexual misconduct that is substantially related to the qualifications, functions or duties of a psychologist or psychological assistant or registered psychologist. (§ 2960[o])

> New revocation statute. If an Administrative Law Judge finds sexual misconduct with patient or former patient where the therapeutic relationship was terminated for the purposes of engaging in sexual contact, then revocation is automatic. (§ 2960[o])

Rule #2: Do not engage in sexual fantasies about your client.

1. It is normal to have sexual fantasies about your clients, but it is improper to encourage yourself to have these fantasies. Often allowing yourself the luxury of your fantasies may normalize them for you, thereby increasing the probability you may act them out.
2. Take charge of your own thoughts and divert them to other topics.
3. Consciously, stop any sexual thinking about a client. If necessary, use the behavioral technique of Thought Stopping.

Rule #3: Do not be involved in any conduct of a sexual nature which would constitute a conflict of interest with a client.

1. This refers to multiple relationships.
2. Do not treat:

   - Former sexual partners
   - Spouses
   - Current sexual partners
   - Likely future sexual partners

3. Do not engage in sexualized behavior such as hugs, back rubs, hand holding, or other physical contact that has a sexual connotation for either you or your client.

Rule #4: Use the conflict of interest analytical model to guide your actions (see Chapter 2).

Rule #5: If you are aware of significant sexual feelings for a client, immediately seek consultation or therapy.

Chapter 5

SEX WITH FORMER
THERAPY CLIENTS

One of the more controversial problems in multiple relationships deals with involvement in sexual contact with former therapy clients. Although the rules in law and ethics are clear regarding sexual contact with current patients, they are much more ambiguous regarding sexual contact with former clients. Many state laws do not prohibit such conduct directly. Several authors have addressed the problems of engaging in posttermination sexual contact with a former patient (Gabbard, 1994; Gabbard & Pope, 1989; Haas & Malouf, 2005; Koocher & Keith-Spiegel, 1998).

Ethics codes are not as direct and specific as they are for sex with current patients. For example, the AAMFT has adopted the 2-year rule; that is, sexual conduct is considered unethical until 2 years after therapy has been terminated (AAMFT, 2001). In addition, the APA adopted a 2-year rule in its 1992 revision of its ethics code (APA, 1992) and in the revised code (APA, 2002). The American Psychiatric Association has the clearest and most strict rule in the mental health profession. The American Psychiatric Association rule is as follows: "Sexual activity with a current or former patient is unethical" (2001, § 2.1).

The American Psychological Association rule is interesting because it does not conclude that sexual contact with a former client is, per se, acceptable after 2 years. The psychologist must justify his or her actions even after waiting for 2 years. The NASW changed its code of ethics to prohibit sexual contact with former therapy clients (NASW, 1999, 1.09[c]). The American Counseling Association was the last professional group to write language prohibiting sex with former clients (ACA, 2005, § A.5.b.). Table 6 (pp. 46-47) presents the language used with regard to sex with former clients by the various associations.

TABLE 6: Sexual Conduct With Former Patients/Clients

American Psychological Association (APA)

§ 10.08 Sexual Intimacies With Former Therapy Clients/Patients

(a) Psychologists do not engage in sexual intimacies with former clients/patients for at least two years after cessation or termination of therapy.

(b) Psychologists do not engage in sexual intimacies with former clients/patients even after a two-year interval except in the most unusual circumstances. Psychologists who engage in such activity after the two years following cessation or termination of therapy and of having no sexual contact with the former client/patient bear the burden of demonstrating that there has been no exploitation, in light of all relevant factors, including (1) the amount of time that has passed since therapy terminated; (2) the nature, duration, and intensity of the therapy; (3) the circumstances of termination; (4) the client's/patient's personal history; (5) the client's/patient's current mental status; (6) the likelihood of adverse impact on the client/patient; and (7) any statements or actions made by the therapist during the course of therapy suggesting or inviting the possibility of a posttermination sexual or romantic relationship with the client/patient.

American Association for Marriage and Family Therapy (AAMFT)

§ 1.5 Sexual intimacy with former clients is likely to be harmful and is therefore prohibited for two years following the termination of therapy or last professional contact.

National Association of Social Workers (NASW)

§ 1.09 (c) Social workers should not engage in sexual activities or sexual contact with former clients because of the potential for harm to the client.

American Psychiatric Association

§ 2.1 Sexual activity with a current or former patient is unethical.

American Counseling Association (ACA)

§ A.5.a. **Current Clients**

Sexual or romantic counselor–client interactions or relationships with current clients, their romantic partners, or their family members are prohibited.

§ A.5.b. **Former Clients**

Sexual or romantic counselor–client interactions or relationships with former clients, their romantic partners, or their family members are prohibited for a period of 5 years following the last professional contact. Counselors, before engaging in sexual or romantic interactions or relationships with clients, their romantic partners, or client family members after 5 years following the last professional contact, demonstrate forethought and document (in written form) whether the interactions or relationship can be viewed as exploitive in some way and/or whether there is still potential to harm the former client; in cases of potential exploitation and/or harm, the counselor avoids entering such an interaction or relationship.

§ F.3.b. **Sexual Relationships**

Sexual or romantic interactions or relationships with current supervisees are prohibited.

American Association of Pastoral Counselors (AAPC)

§ III.H We recognize that the therapist/client relationship involves a power imbalance, the residual effects of which are operative following the termination of the therapy relationship. Therefore, all sexual behavior or harassment as defined in Principle III, G with former clients is unethical.

This ambiguity is likely to create confusion in the therapist who is required to live by such rules. Although the APA, ACA, NASW, and AAMFT have adopted a 2-year rule, not every professional organization has followed this pattern, and ethics writers generally oppose setting any time period as a marker for acceptable professional-client sex. The American Psychiatric Association clearly prohibits sexual contact with former clients. The AAPC creates a strict rule consistent with the American Psychiatric Association and rejects the 2-year rule. But what is the significance of 2 years? Gabbard (1994) addresses the arguments in favor of any sexual contact with a former patient at any time. Gabbard's analysis of the arguments is quite compelling and leaves one to conclude that there is no justification for engaging in sexual contact with a former therapy client.

There are six compelling arguments against having sexual contact with a former client: The first is that it is difficult, if not impossible, for the client to perceive the therapist as anything but a former therapist. Gabbard (1994) refers to this as the internalized therapist. The therapist-client relationship is so strong, powerful, and influential that it does not dissipate after 2 years. Many relationships are similar. Haas and Malouf (2005) recommend the "once a client, always a client" standard.

As an example in my teachings, one question I ask my students is to think of your sixth-grade teacher. Is there any way you can think about your sixth-grade teacher other than as your sixth-grade teacher? To this day I can imagine Sister Ann Laura, my sixth-grade teacher, who, in my mind, is still my teacher from that era; this is 31 years later. For those therapists who have been in therapy, do you not still think of your former therapist as your therapist?

Second, the power that exists in the therapy relationship that is ultimately useful in assisting clients through difficult issues lingers on long after therapy has ceased. This differential power creates an uneven balance between the former therapist and the former patient long after therapy has been terminated. This power, as well as the perception of the therapy relationship, is still extant after termination and may last a lifetime.

The problem with the differential level of power is that it may cause a former patient to agree to enter into a personal relationship with a former therapist based upon the abuse of the power and not truly based upon free will. Hence, in the present, the therapist would be taking advantage of the former role as a therapist to gain personally with the former client.

Third, Gabbard (1994) also correctly concludes that there may be a continuing professional relationship after the termination of therapy.

There may be posttermination contact pertaining to legal action, records, and consultation. Many clients return for therapy years later.

Fourth, there is evidence that posttermination sexual contact may harm the patient, thereby undoing what was accomplished in treatment.

Fifth, the therapy process itself may be harmed, not only for the patient, but for those who are contemplating entering into treatment but choose not to because they learn of posttermination sexual contact between a therapist and a former patient.

A final reason against engaging in sexual contact with a former patient is that it almost assuredly precludes a patient from returning to treatment with the therapist. It is very common for patients to terminate therapy, only to enter treatment elsewhere at a later time. Engaging in a personal relationship is likely to prohibit the patient from returning to therapy, thereby depriving him or her of the privilege of seeking treatment from a safe, reliable, predictable, and helpful therapist who has a proven track record of providing valuable assistance.

One of the most fascinating cases to be litigated to the appellate level was *Poliak v. Board of Psychology* (1997). This case involved allegations of sexualized therapy and subsequent sexual conduct after therapy had been terminated. The Third District Court of Appeals in California reversed the decision of the California Board of Psychology to revoke the license of Dr. Poliak, who engaged in sexual contact with a former client. The reversal was based on an error in the charging document referring to the former patient as a "patient," which implied that the individual was still in therapy. In other cases, however, mental health professionals have actually faced disciplinary action, often by settlement, with various state licensing boards. In other words, the *Poliak* case stands out as a unique legal matter which was decided on a technicality in the charging document. To my knowledge, the California Boards have never made such a mistake again. There is no other case similar to Poliak where a licensing board made an error in their charging document regarding sexual behavior with a former client.

Reasons to Engage in Sexual Contact With a Former Client

1. You may encounter a former client, incidentally, when there has not been contact for many years, and you still may be attracted to each other because of legitimate changes each of you have made.

2. Your former client may have become a professional therapist and be in contact with you years later through professional meetings and other activities.

Engaging in sexual conduct with a former client is very risky. The APA *Ethical Principles and Code of Conduct* (APA, 2002) sets forth several considerations that must be analyzed before sexual behavior with a former patient might not be considered unethical. In fact, engaging in sexual conduct is probably never truly ethical. Further, licensing boards across the country seem split on whether such conduct may be actionable. For example, after much debate, California settled on a 2-year rule (Ca. Civil Code § 43.93). The fact that there is a differential level of power between a former patient and a therapist may be sufficient to vitiate consent. Be extremely cautious with severely disturbed individuals, because they may not be competent to give consent. In such a situation the former therapist could be charged with rape or another very serious sexual offense.

Reasons Not to Engage in Sexual Contact With a Former Client

1. It may be extremely harmful to the former client.
2. Many former clients who may have been victims of prior sexual abuse may become involved in sexual conduct with their therapists. It too is a form of revictimization.
3. It may be a violation of the professional licensing laws established in the United States and can result in revocation of one's license, depending upon the circumstances.
4. It is a violation of the professional ethics code of all mental health professionals and can result in expulsion from a professional association.
5. It may be an indication of impairment on the part of the therapist.
6. Former patients who were victims of therapist abuse may engage in sexualized behavior in hopes that a safe therapist will not take advantage of them.
7. It is harmful to the public's perception of the profession of mental health and may hinder others from entering into therapy.
8. In several states it constitutes criminal conduct and can result in a jail sentence.

9. If the former client does not have the capacity to consent to the sexual conduct, your conduct will be considered a felony.
10. It is prohibited for psychiatrists and pastoral counselors.
11. There is a 2-year rule in effect for psychologists, social workers, counselors, and marriage and family therapists.

Circumstances in Which it Is Acceptable to Have Contact With a Former Client

1. There has not been any contact for a period of 5 years or more.
2. The nature of the professional service was short term and somewhat impersonal.
3. The contact that led to entering into a relationship with a former client years later was unplanned, incidental, and serendipitous.
4. The former client is a psychologically healthy individual with the full capacity to consent.
5. The professional is psychologically healthy and not in a particularly vulnerable mental state.
6. An objective legal and mental health consultant has agreed that the conduct is not prohibited and may be acceptable.
7. You live in a rural area.
8. There are no state laws that prohibit your conduct.

All of the above-listed eight factors must apply for a professional to consider entering into a sexual relationship with a former client. I do not condone sexual contact with a former client. It is my belief that it is always unwise and, most likely, always unethical. Consequently, I adhere to the "once a client, always a client" point of view that has emerged in the past 15 years.

Rules for Professional Practice

Rule # 1: Do not have sexual contact with a former patient—ever!

Rule # 2: If you do decide to have sexual contact with a former patient, wait for a period of 5 years, determine that you have a good reason for the sexual contact, be in a position to demonstrate there has not been contact with the former patient for the previous 5 years, and meet the former client only incidentally. In addition, all eight factors noted previously must apply.

Rule #3: Seek consultation prior to engaging in sexual contact with a former patient after the 2-year, preferably 5-year, waiting period.

Rule #4: If your consultant agrees that sexual contact with a former client is ethical, consult with an objective legal and mental health consultant and seek a third opinion from another objective consultant.

Rule #5: Be very certain your former client is competent to consent to sexual contact with you.

Chapter 6

SEX AND OTHER MULTIPLE RELATIONSHIPS WITH STUDENTS AND SUPERVISEES

During the past 15 years there has been increasing concern regarding personal relationships with students and supervisees. The future career of a student or a supervisee is often in the hands of one person. The student or supervisee may feel that his or her ability to make free choices is constrained because the professor or supervisor has so much power and control over him or her. Rules regarding protection of students and supervisees are essentially universal among the major ethical codes of mental health professions, but are also relatively recent. Authors have noted that students and supervisees are often very dependent upon the approval of a supervisor or teacher. Their entire future as a mental health professional may depend upon the approval, reference, or passing grade of a teacher or supervisor.

A graduate student working on his or her dissertation under a professor is in a highly vulnerable position in the relationship. This vulnerability translates into a need to please the instructor and to acquiesce to the needs of the professor. Differential power is present to a great extent in both supervisor-supervisee and student-teacher relationships. That is, the supervisor and teacher have greater levels of power in their relationships with their students and supervisors which could lead to misuse of that power. From a standpoint of harm, a vulnerable student or supervisee could suffer great harm if his or her true needs are not taken into account and if the supervisor does not choose to act virtuously to assist the individual in his or her rite of passage into the profession. The virtuous teacher has a great opportunity to model the judicious use of differential power in a relationship, similar to what happens in therapy relationships and other relationships involving the provision of psychological services. This commitment to virtue is now more important in the training of future professionals than actual knowledge. We know from research on abuse that the abused often become abusers when they grow up. The damaged individual often goes on to damage others; those taken advantage of will learn how to do so to others. This problem has been commented upon by many authors (Koocher & Keith-Spiegel, 1998; Kurpius et al., 1991; Miller & Larrabee, 1995; Newman, 1981). Probably the most detailed code of ethics dealing with supervisor-supervisee relationships was developed by the American Association for Counseling and Development (AACD, 1988). Items that have not been fully addressed are the specific prohibitions, the timing of such prohibitions, and the most important reason to control impulses and act virtuously in supervisory relationships, whether the recipient is a student or a supervisee. Modeling appropriate behavior has been considered one of the primary duties of the supervisor (Allen, Szollos, & Williams, 1986). Recent publications suggest that ethicists are taking a closer look at the problems associated with multiple relationships between students and teachers (Blevins-Knabe, 2003; Slimp & Burian, 2003). These authors are highly critical of sexual relationships between students and professors.

Sex With Students
And Supervisees

Anyone who trained in mental health in the 1970s and 1980s became aware of numerous cases of sexual relations between professors and students and between supervisors and supervisees. Several professional organizations have developed specific rules prohibiting sexual conduct between a teacher and a student (APA, 2002, §7.07; ACA, 2005, § F.3.; AAMFT, 2001, § 4.3; NASW, 1999, § 2.07; AAPC, 1994, § V). See Table 7 (pp. 56-57) for the language used with regard to sex with students and supervisees by the various associations. Many people are aware of professors who engaged in sexual contact with multiple students or supervisees. In the 1970s, one college professor told me, "I want to have sex with as many of my students as possible." This particular person carried out his goal and was notorious, but no adverse action was taken against him. There have been recent cases of supervisors being disciplined by licensing boards for engaging in sexual misconduct with supervisees, including a case where the supervisor engaged in inappropriate conduct with two of his supervisees (see *In the Matter of the Accusation Against Larry A. Nadig*, 1992). In this case, Dr. Nadig's license was revoked, but the revocation was stayed and he received 6 years of intensive probation.

The American Psychological Association recognized that students and supervisees were subject to sexual exploitation (APA, 2002; Knapp & Vandecreek, 2003). Allen et al. (1986) noted the similarity between the relationship of therapist and patient and that of supervisor and supervisee. The American Counseling Association recognizes the unique relationship extant between a student and a teacher. Consequently, they promulgated rules to prevent such exploitation (ACA, 2005). The real issue is that a supervisee or student may consent to engage in sexual conduct with a teacher or supervisor, not because it is their free and voluntary choice to do so, but because they feel they have no choice and must provide sexual favors to pass a course, complete a degree program, have a dissertation approved, or have hours of training signed off by the supervisor or teacher. This lack of free choice created by the relationship is part of the problem. The dynamics of relationships serve to vitiate consent and choice, to some degree. Lack of true choice in sexual relations is a problem likely to result in psychological damage to the person who, in effect, consents under obvious or subtle duress. Hence, sexual contact between supervisors and supervisees should be considered unethical and a serious breach of the standard of care. Further, sexual contact between a teacher and a student while the student is in a class or in a formal training relationship with the teacher should also be considered unethical. Although there may be times when a student or supervisee will truly make a free choice to engage in a relationship with a teacher or supervisor, the likelihood of exploitation is so great as to argue against any type of sexual relationship while there is a primary professional relationship in existence.

The strongest argument in support of such a prohibition is that of virtuous modeling. The students/supervisees are learning a profession, which means that they are becoming a different type of person: individuals who will integrate ideas, methods, a style of thinking, a manner of being, and ethical responsibility toward others into their personalities, if training is successful. They must be taught through didactic and experiential means. The instructors must model appropriate behavior, including how to deal with sexual attraction and how to control sexual impulses. In the training of mental health professionals, this lesson is one of the most important, given the fact that sexual misconduct is the single most common cause for disciplinary action for mental health professionals (Association of State and Provincial Psychology Boards [ASPPB], 1997).

In a teaching situation, the professor has the power to pass or fail the student. The student could receive honors recognition for work in the class or no recognition whatsoever. The student is in somewhat of

TABLE 7: Sexual Conduct With Students or Supervisees

American Psychological Association (APA)

§ 7.07   Sexual Relationships With Students and Supervisees

Psychologists do not engage in sexual relationships with students or supervisees who are in their department, agency, or training center or over whom psychologists have or are likely to have evaluative authority.

American Association for Marriage and Family Therapy (AAMFT)

§ 4.1   Marriage and family therapists are aware of their influential positions with respect to students and supervisees, and they avoid exploiting the trust and dependency of such persons.

§ 4.3   Marriage and family therapists do not engage in sexual intimacy with students or supervisees during the evaluative or training relationship between the therapist and student or supervisee.

National Association of Social Workers (NASW)

§ 2.07   (a) Social workers who function as supervisors or educators should not engage in sexual activities or contact with supervisees, students, trainees, or other colleagues over whom they exercise professional authority.

§ 3.01   (b) Social workers who provide supervision or consultation are responsible for setting clear, appropriate, and culturally sensitive boundaries.

        (c) Social workers should not engage in any dual or multiple relationships with supervisees in which there is a risk of exploitation of or potential harm to the supervisee.

American Psychiatric Association

§ 4.14   Sexual involvement between faculty member or supervisor and a trainee or student, in those situations in which an abuse of power can occur, often takes advantage of inequalities in the working relationship and may be unethical because:

    a.   Any treatment of a patient being supervised may be deleteriously affected.

    b.   It may damage the trust relationship between teacher and student.

    c.   Teachers are important professional role models for their trainees and affect their trainee's future professional behavior.

American Counseling Association (ACA)

§ F.3.a. Relationship Boundaries With Supervisees

Counseling supervisors clearly define and maintain ethical professional, personal, and social relationships with their supervisees. Counseling supervisors avoid nonprofessional relationships with current supervisees. If supervisors must assume other professional roles (e.g., clinical and administrative supervisor, instructor) with supervisees, they work to minimize potential conflicts and explain to supervisees the expectations and responsibilities associated with each role. They do not engage in any form of nonprofessional interaction that may compromise the supervisory relationship.

§ F.3.b. Sexual Relationships

Sexual or romantic interactions or relationships with current supervisees are prohibited.

§ F.10.a. Sexual or Romantic Relationships

Sexual or romantic interactions or relationships with current students are prohibited.

§ F.10.c. Relationships With Former Students

Counselor educators are aware of the power differential in the relationship between faculty and students. Faculty members foster open discussions with former students when considering engaging in a social, sexual, or other intimate relationship. Faculty members discuss with the former student how their former relationship may affect the change in relationship.

American Association of Pastoral Counselors (AAPC)

§ V.B.

We do not engage in sexual or other harassment of supervisees, students, employees, research subjects or colleagues.

a vulnerable position, although not nearly as vulnerable as a psycho-therapy patient. Often professors are revered by their students, in part because they have knowledge of a subject of interest for the student, and also because the professor is at the center of attention for months. Further, the professor is an authority figure who is often placed in high esteem by the student. The student's perception of the professor as a powerful authority object creates an atmosphere in which exploitation could occur. The professor might take advantage of the student's perception to have the student consent to engage in sexual rela-tions with the professor, where he or she otherwise would not. The consent occurs not as a truly free choice but as the result of the duplicitous behavior of the professor coupled with the vulnerability of the student. Likewise, student-teacher relationships that extend across a longer period of time, such as when the student is writing a dissertation under a professor, are more problematic in that the con-sequences for not acquiescing to the requests of the professor are much more onerous. These consequences might include rejection of the entire dissertation, resulting in the student being unable to gradu-ate and enter a chosen profession.

Likewise, a supervisor of a psychological intern is also in a posi-tion of trust and authority. Often the supervisor meets with the trainee on a day-to-day basis. The trainee must accrue creditable hours in order to complete an internship, residency, or supervision hours required for licensure.

The supervisor has the power, in some instances, to reject a year's worth of work of the trainee. The stakes are very high for the trainee, who might agree to enter into a personal relationship with the supervisor, fearing that not to do so could jeopardize securing the needed hours and experience necessary for licensure. Several supervisors have taken advantage of their position of authority in this manner. Many supervisors who acted out their sexual impulses were not predators but were actually infatuated with their supervisees. Nevertheless, the results often are harmful to the trainee. Further, the personal relationship is likely to impede the objectivity of the professor or supervisor, potentially leading to ineffectiveness of the process.

Currently no express prohibitions exist against sexual conduct with a former student or supervisee. One reason is that the relationship is not as intense as it is in a psychotherapy setting; the power of the supervisor/professor is greatly diminished after the formal supervisor-supervisee relationship has ended and the need for continued objectivity is no longer present. Further, a diminution in objectivity caused by the personal relationship is not particularly significant once the teaching or supervisory relationship has ended. In deciding to enter into a personal relationship with a former supervisee or student, the following factors should be considered:

1. Has the primary relationship been terminated for the purpose of entering into a personal relationship? If so, the personal relationship should not occur.
2. Has there been a reasonable length of time between the professional relationship and the personal one? Consider a minimum of a few months.
3. What is the likelihood of reestablishing a professional relationship in the future? If there is a chance of a future professional relationship, then no personal relationship should occur.
4. Does the student or supervisee have any particular vulnerabilities that might allow him or her to become involved in a personal relationship with the professor or supervisor? These could take the form of mental disorders, prior abuse by an authority figure, the lack of other prior relationships with people, or some unique characteristic of the student/supervisee.
5. Is there anything about the personal relationship that might cause significant harm to the student/supervisee?
6. Is the relationship occurring by the free will of both parties?
7. Has an objective consultant been unable to identify any reasons not to enter into the proposed relationship?
8. What was the length of time of the professional relationship? The greater the time of the professional relationship, the greater the care required by the professor or supervisee.
9. Has anyone voiced a valid concern about the potential future personal relationship? This concern could come from a friend, colleague, therapist, licensing board member, or faculty member.

These considerations will lead to well-reasoned behavior by the supervisor or the professor.

Socializing With Students and Supervisees

Currently, no rules exist in any mental health ethics code or in any state law that prohibit a supervisor from socializing with a student. In fact, healthy social interaction may be a positive experience for all involved and may be instructive as well. Social contact with students and supervisees should be encouraged, provided it is appropriate, nonexploitative, and nonharmful. This means that the supervisor/ professor has an affirmative duty to maintain proper decorum. Consider the following example:

> T. Cher, PhD, is a full professor at the University of High Honors. She has taught there for the past 20 years. One of the classes she teaches is advanced systems theory in psychology with advanced PhD students. Every Friday night she meets her class at the Red Herring Bar & Grill for dinner and a few drinks. They use the time to talk about the world, their personal lives, and psychology in general. Students who have graduated have all reported fondly on these extracurricular sessions. Dr. Cher, while consuming a few drinks, had never become intoxicated in any of the out-of-class sessions, and none of these sessions led to a sexual relationship with a student.

This example demonstrates a social activity not atypical of what many teachers and students consider a central part of learning. The teacher conducts herself appropriately and within the parameters of her role. She does not use the social experience to her benefit by exploiting students, nor does any obvious harm flow from the experience. Often the complete learning experience in graduate training involves close interactions with the professors, both inside and outside the classroom. Would it matter in the example noted above if Dr. Cher hosted her students at her house, or if she served them wine in moderation, or participated with them in an exercise such as running, softball, tennis, golf, basketball, darts, bowling, soccer, la crosse, or met with them at a student's home? Most likely not, because the basic role characteristics are in place and Dr. Cher is in no way using her position of authority to gain an undue advantage over her students.

What if Dr. Cher went dancing with her students or used drugs with them, such as cocaine, methamphetamine, marijuana, or LSD? The answer is logically derived from the parameters set forth above. Clearly, going dancing, without additional facts, is acceptable, while using drugs is unacceptable. The use of illicit substances is not consistent with a role model who is teaching adherence to societal rules. Engaging in illegal activity is generally not an appropriate social activity in which to participate with students, just like robbing a bank or breaking windows in the school administration building would be totally inappropriate. But could there be unlawful activities that follow a social relationship with a teacher that may be appropriate? If one accepts the idea of universally based ethical principles, then it may be necessary to engage in some unlawful activities; there may be a fundamental duty to do so. Consider those mental health professionals who have worked in repressive political regimes where political dissidents have been committed to psychiatric facilities or where freedoms of individual choice, speech, association, and privacy have been completely eliminated, or where people are tortured or held without a valid reason. In these and similar circumstances there may be a duty to do all that is necessary to promote the individual and societal rights that the founding fathers and mothers of the United States considered inalienable and that many, if not all, religious groups espouse to some degree or another.

Most socialization is probably both acceptable and ethical. In fact, positive socialization with impulse control should not be feared but should be encouraged. Likewise, the examples used above for students all apply to supervisees in that the supervisee is in a slightly stronger position of power. Social activities that should be considered appropriate include:

1. Breakfast, lunch, snacks, and dinner
2. Playing or attending sporting events
3. Visiting museums, monuments, historic sites
4. Socializing in the home of the teacher/supervisor or student
5. Picnics
6. Camping trips
7. Travel, including longer trips
8. Attending an important event of the student/supervisee, such as a wedding, bar mitzvah, graduation, birthday party, and so on
9. Driving together to places
10. Taking walks

As long as the primary relationship is maintained, it would seem appropriate to socialize. Some might argue that the teacher/supervisor should maintain strict boundaries with students/supervisees in order to model appropriate role behavior which will eventually be applied to dealing with patients. However, in a criminal case that took place in 2004, an Air Force officer used camping trips with his supervisees to take advantage of them sexually. This individual was sent to prison for 10 years (*U. S. v. Fujiwara*, 2004). Clinical supervisors should put the primary focus on modeling appropriate behavior and maintaining boundaries with their patients. Teachers who provide treatment can do the same with their students. One of the subtleties of learning is to teach students to discriminate among complex variables, making appropriate clinical and behavioral choices while avoiding rationalizations. There is a very delicate yet important distinction between rationalization and discriminating thought. The student is to gain knowledge, apply the knowledge to factual circumstances, learn when to discriminate and when to generalize, and to limit rationalizing to a minimum.

Financial Dealings
With Students and Supervisees

There have been numerous stories and actual cases involving teachers and supervisors who borrowed money or entered into business relationships with students/supervisees. In one unpublished case, a teacher at a school who was also an administrator borrowed thousands of dollars from his students without his supervisors knowing about it. It was only after he failed to pay them back that the students complained and the teacher was fired. Problems with repayment result in bad feelings, complaints against the borrower, and often deeply irreparable perceptions about the profession. It is quite different to borrow 75 cents for a glass of soda or even a few dollars for lunch than it is to borrow a few thousand dollars. The difference in this case is the amount, and the amount is relevant to the analysis of whether it constitutes a conflict of interest. This is because there is no absolute expressed prohibition. The rules requiring nonexploitation and no harm to students and supervisors apply. From these rules comes the essential guidance requiring due care in the actions of the teacher/supervisor toward the student/supervisee.

Although there is no actual dollar amount written in any ethics textbook beyond which constitutes exploitation, there is some guidance in other areas. The Fair Political Practices Commission in California requires the recording and reporting of any gift greater than $250 by a governmental official (CA Government Code § 89503, 2001). Other rules set forth a $25 figure, which is more appropriate for mental health professionals. This figure has been selected somewhat arbitrarily, although it is based upon the study of gifts to legislators and other members of government. A gift of less than $25 is considered insignificant. Anything more is considered suspect. The teacher or supervisor who uses the $25 figure will not likely have a problem, especially if the teacher pays the student/supervisee back. Although it is safest not to borrow any money, a small amount which is paid back immediately is probably not a conflict, nor would it be any type of a major ethical problem.

Business Ventures

Few students enter into business ventures with their teachers, although it is not unusual for a former teacher to enter a business with a former student such as practicing therapy together in a group practice. Fortunately it is a limited number, because it is not ethical to have a business relationship with a teacher. There are likely to be significant conflicts in such relationships. It is not uncommon for supervisors to enter into business relations with their supervisees. The most common form of a business relationship is paying for supervision. This type of transaction has been debated by state licensing boards and experts in ethics. Some experts believe it is a conflict as well as a dual relationship to pay for supervision. In California, supervisees are prohibited from paying for supervision (Ca. Code of Regulations, Title 16 § 1387 et seq., 2001). However, in other states, such as in Iowa, it is perfectly legal for a supervisor to charge for supervision. There is no clear agreement among state licensing boards about this issue. Further, there is no guidance in any mental health ethics code. However, the basic rules of nonexploitation and no harm apply. Hence, the amount of the charge is always going to be relevant to a determination of whether the conduct was ethical and appropriate. A charge of $500 per hour undoubtedly will be viewed as exploitative in 2006, while a charge of $80 would be considered reasonable.

The second most common business relationship between the supervisor and supervisee is where the supervisee has an interest in the professional property where patients are seen; often this is in the form of a leasehold. In some cases the supervisee actually owns the property or is the primary leaseholder. In other cases the supervisor and supervisee are both leaseholders. This creates an inherent conflict of interest, especially if the supervisee is the owner or primary lessee. As owner, the supervisee has a distinct business relationship with the supervisor. Typically, an owner can terminate the lease under certain conditions, take legal action to evict a tenant, and is responsible for repairs on the property. A dispute between a supervisor and supervisee could expand to an entirely different and more destructive level for patients and the parties in situations where the supervisee has an interest in the property.

In a few cases the supervisor leases space to the supervisee. This is less problematic but can evolve into a potential problem in that it adds a secondary relationship to the primary professional one, which could create difficulties in and of itself in the supervisory relationship, which is very important and complex. The easiest way to deal with the situation is to make sure the supervisor is the primary leaseholder of the professional office property and be certain the owner is not the supervisee. Further, the supervisee should not pay rent at the office. It is common that a fee for administrative costs is deducted from the charges of the supervisee to patients. There is no law or ethics code provision precluding this practice.

The final way supervisees typically get involved with their supervisors is after the completion of training. Some supervisees choose to enter the practice of their supervisors once the supervisee is fully licensed to practice at the independent level. Other than the guiding principles of nonexploitation and no harm, there is no rule that makes this action unethical or improper. The reason it is proper is that the supervisee is now independent and is not dependent upon the approval or signature of the supervisor. The supervisee is on an equal level with the supervisor. These kinds of relationships should be encouraged, because it means that professionals of like interests are practicing together, potentially exploring new methods of dealing with human problems and advancing the profession. There is no state law or ethics code provision that prevents a supervisee from entering into a business relationship with a former supervisor after the supervisory relationship has been terminated.

Reasons Why One Might Rationalize Engaging in a Sexual Relationship With a Student or Supervisee

1. The supervisor or professor is interested in satisfying his or her own personal needs without regard to the possible effect it may have on the student or supervisee.
2. There may be a genuine attraction between the student/supervisee and the teacher/supervisor.
3. The teacher or supervisor has chosen to ignore ethical and legal constraints.

In actuality, there is no appropriate ethical, legal, or moral reason for a teacher or supervisor to engage in a sexual relationship. Consequently, a professor should not develop his or her dating pool from his or her students.

Reasons Not to Engage in a Sexual Relationship With a Student or Supervisee

1. It is likely to cause harm to the student/supervisee.
2. It will likely impair the objectivity of the relationship.
3. It is bad modeling.
4. It is perceived negatively by the general public and may, therefore, adversely affect the profession.

Rules

Rule #1: Do not engage in a sexual relationship with a student or supervisee.

Rule #2: Wait a minimum of 6 months after the professional relationship has ended to enter into a personal relationship. There must not be a chance that the supervisor or teacher will ever be in the same professional relationship again.

Rule #3: Never end a professional relationship for the purpose of entering into a personal relationship with a student/supervisee.

Rule #4: Always consider the modeling component of conduct in a supervisory/teaching relationship.

Rule #5: Never exploit a student/supervisee by entering into a business relationship with him or her, or using his or her personal property.

Rule #6: Socializing with a student or supervisee is not unethical provided the professional relationship is always kept in mind.

Rule #7: Do not borrow money from a student or supervisee.

Rule #8: If a supervisor does borrow money from a student or supervisee, it should be less than $5 and paid back immediately.

Chapter 7

SOCIAL CONTACT WITH CLIENTS

Many professional ethicists believe that no socialization with clients is appropriate, in part because therapeutic boundaries are blurred, at least theoretically, when this occurs. Some mental health professionals (Borys, 1992; Gabbard, 1994) believe that no social contact is appropriate. However, there are no absolute rules in any ethics codes which prohibit social contact with a client per se. Hence, contact such as lunches, breakfasts, dinners, attending parties, attending meetings, involvement in sports, clubs, or groups, shopping together, driving in the same vehicle together, going to a sporting event with a client, telephone contact outside of therapy, visiting a patient at his or her home, incidental contacts, going to special events of the client such as a wedding or a funeral, as examples, must be limited to unique circumstances and those for which the professional has sought objective consultation. Some social contact may be minimal, such as walking with your client, or the contact may be more extended, such as taking your client to a museum, art gallery, or a special event like a concert or a speech by someone important.

§ A.5.d. Potentially Beneficial Interactions
When a counselor-client nonprofessional interaction with a client or former client may be potentially beneficial to the client or former client, the counselor must document in case records, prior to the interaction (when feasible), the rationale for such an interaction, the potential benefit, and anticipated consequences for the client or former client and other individuals significantly involved with the client or former client. Such interactions should be initiated with appropriate client consent. Where unintentional harm occurs to the client or former client, or to an individual significantly involved with the client or former client, due to the nonprofessional interaction, the counselor must show

evidence of an attempt to remedy such harm. Examples of potentially beneficial interactions include, but are not limited to, attending a formal ceremony (e.g., a wedding/commitment ceremony or graduation); purchasing a service or product provided by a client or former client (excepting unrestricted bartering); hospital visits to an ill family member; mutual membership in a professional association, organization, or community. *(See A.5.c.)* (ACA, 2005)

Further, this is an area in which there are different rules depending upon the nature of the professional relationship. That is, it may actually be beneficial for teachers, supervisors, and consultants to socialize together, while there are more restrictions if there is a therapeutic relationship or if a professional performed an independent evaluation of an individual, such as in the case of worker's compensation, custody, or a court-ordered examination. There is a clear benefit for a supervisor or a teacher to interact socially with his or her students and supervisees, although there is no benefit for the student to have sex with his or her supervisor or teacher. This is an example of the prohibited class of behavior versus conduct that is not prohibited per se.

Various Social Contacts

Therapist Socialization

It is clear that therapists often socialize with their clients. In fact, Borys and Pope (1989) found that 38.8% of therapists found it "ethical under some conditions" (p. 286) and had some potential prior knowledge of or social contact with their clients. Is socializing always unethical? The answer must be a resounding no, or, more precisely, it depends. This is where the harm and interest analysis is helpful. I am hesitant to write about the ambiguity of the rules that exist, because therapists who are impaired in some way will rationalize why they acted improperly in a given situation. This part of the book is not designed to create fuel for the rationalization of impaired therapists; rather, it is designed to create fuel for the reasoning process to be applied by ethical, psychologically healthy therapists.

Breakfast or Lunch

If a therapist goes to breakfast or lunch with a client as a measure of support, assuming the therapist is not impaired or the client so disturbed as to misinterpret the experience, there is no ethical prohibition in this act. It may even be helpful to the client. This presumes that the lunch is in a nonintimate setting and that no alcohol or other psychoactive substances are consumed. A lunch with a client may be helpful to mark an anniversary or a significant step in therapy, provide needed external support to the client, or demonstrate acceptance of the client. It may occur to mark the termination point in therapy. However, it must occur with the client's best interest in mind, not the therapist's interest. It must also be infrequent. The frequency of the social activity can support or cloud the therapeutic boundaries. There is no scientific evidence that an infrequent lunch with a client in which therapeutic parameters are maintained is harmful. However, some research suggests that any activity which promotes the interests of the therapist to the detriment of the client and is frequent may blur therapeutic boundaries. This is a critically important issue because the relationship is the tool used in most therapies. As previously stated, some have made the analogy that those who blur therapeutic boundaries are similar to surgeons who allow their scalpels to become contaminated with bacteria.

A lunch with a client to mark or celebrate termination is clearly not unethical per se. A lunch with a client during the midst of therapy, with a borderline client, which is intimate in nature and set up because the therapist is feeling lonely, is a serious problem and will, in all likelihood, lead to additional boundary violations.

But what about the situation in which you are invited to a special luncheon celebrating a major ethnic holiday or a special family event? Would this not be in the interests of the client to attend? Further, there would be no aura of intimacy. It may be culturally appropriate to attend and may be an insult not to go.

Again, issues such as frequency of the lunches, the intimacy of the setting, the framing of the event, the psychological health of the therapist and client, the theoretical orientation of the therapist, and the nature of the event itself must be taken into account. In the military, for example, medical personnel who work with flight crews are expected to interact with the crews on and off the job. Those medical and psychological personnel who do not interact with wing personnel are not visited voluntarily by these individuals. Hence, a person who genuinely needs treatment may not seek it because of the therapeutic boundaries and rules being interpreted too strictly. This is a case of the social culture dictating and affecting the ethical rules of practice. It also depends upon whether the activity—in this case, a lunch—is considered appropriate given the theoretical model of the therapist. Therapists who are psychoanalytic or psychodynamic often treat patients for years. A significant aspect of this long-term therapy is the purity of the relationship. Extratherapeutic contact is discouraged in these models.

Other factors that must be considered are the psychological health of the therapist, the psychological state of the client, and the number of people (witnesses) who will observe the lunch. The poorer the psychological health of the therapist or the patient, the greater the likelihood for a problem to develop, even with lunch.

Dinner

Going to dinner with a client is much more complicated. The author recalls going to dinner with a group of individuals who attended an assertiveness training program. The dinner occurred at the last class session and was a test of assertiveness at the restaurant. Clearly that type of contact is ethical and in the interests of the clients. It was a group activity. But what about a private dinner with an individual therapy client? One must first ask, "Why am I going to dinner with a client?" If the answer leads to a conclusion that your own needs are being met by the activity and/or there is a sexual connotation, then the activity is clearly inappropriate. It is always important to keep in mind the factors that make the activity unethical. Those factors are harm, exploitation, and impairment in the parties or the relationship, and they can cause a lack of objectivity, create confusion for the client or therapist, or be perceived as unethical. Finally, prior to engaging in such activity the professional should obtain clearance from an independent and objective consultant (see Appendix C on pages 173-174 for guidelines on choosing a consultant).

In most circumstances this may give the client the idea that something more intimate than a therapeutic relationship exists between the client and the therapist. Going to dinner with a client may create a conflict of interest; it may very well be unethical. It also may be the beginning of a problem.

The therapist should always assess the motive for the activity. Using the decision-making model, the motive for the activity clearly should be to promote the interests of the client and not those of the therapist. As noted above, the client and therapist should be of sufficient psychological health to understand that therapeutic boundaries exist despite the fact that the contact is taking place outside a therapy office. A therapist should never go to dinner with a patient who has a Borderline, Histrionic, Paranoid, or Schizotypal Personality Disorder, nor should the therapist go to dinner with a client who has a Dissociative Identity Disorder or a Bipolar Disorder in a manic phase, a psychotic patient, or a schizophrenic, unless the activity is a planned, structured outing as part of a treatment center with several staff members present. Any dinner with a particular client that occurs more than once should raise serious questions for the therapist. The therapist must examine why a particular client has been selected to go to dinner. The therapist must consider the following factors:

1. The purpose of the activity.
2. What needs of the client are being met by the dinner.
3. What needs of the therapist are met by the dinner.
4. Whether any sexual overtones are present.
5. What the therapist's independent consultant has advised about the activity.
6. Whether the therapist is vulnerable to act out in other ways with this client.

Parties

Should you ever attend a party that a client of yours will be attending? The answer is, it depends. There is no absolute proscription against attending a party where a client is present. No ethical code has specifically prohibited such an activity. Further, there is no published ethics case in which a mental health professional was punished for attending a party with a client. There are those who would consider such an activity inappropriate and probably unethical (Borys, 1992). No one would require a therapist to leave a party where a client appeared without the therapist's prior knowledge. But what about the circumstance where a party has been planned and the therapist is fully aware the client will be attending? There are some things to consider when deciding whether to attend a party under the preceding circumstances. It is important to consider:

1. Where the party will be held—at the home of the therapist or the home of a mutual friend or acquaintance.
2. The number of people who will be attending the party (the smaller the attendance, the greater the likelihood of a problem developing).
3. The reason for the party.
4. The formality of the event.
5. The intimacy of the event.
6. The likelihood that illicit substances may be present.
7. The likelihood that significant alcohol consumption will be encouraged.
8. The reason for the attendance of the therapist.
9. The physical time of the party.
10. Whether there is any sexual connotation attached to the therapist's attendance at the party.

11. Whether the therapist will be attending the event in the role of a therapist.
12. The nature of the specific role of the client.
13. Whether this has ever occurred before or if this would be an exception to a long-standing practice against such conduct.
14. Whether the therapist believes there is something special about the person versus something special about the situation that leads to a decision to attend. (If the therapist rationalizes to the extent that he or she determines something is special about the person, then extra caution should be exercised to the extent that the therapist should probably not attend the function. If the event is special, such as a graduation, retirement, recovery from an illness, baby shower, receipt of an award, wedding, funeral, or other recognized important event, then it may be acceptable to attend. Thinking a patient is special could be a warning sign that the therapist's feelings are rising to the extent they may impair judgment and impede rationality.)

In addition to the above factors that must be considered, the therapist must conduct the harm and conflict analysis prior to going to the event in question. In addition, there are specific considerations regarding parties. One consideration is where the party is being held. A party held at the home of the therapist or the client should immediately be viewed as suspicious. That is, the therapist should not attend a party at a client's home or have the client attend a party at his or her home unless a good reason exists. There may be a good reason to attend a party at the home of a client. A client who is having a graduation party celebrating his or her graduation from college may be an appropriate event for the therapist to attend briefly, provided the motive for attendance is to promote the interests of the client in some way, such as celebrating this rite of passage in a very professional manner. The therapist would continue to operate in the role of therapist and not in a different capacity.

The ethics codes of all professional organizations have general rules applicable to dual relationships (see Table 1, pp. 6-8).

It may be appropriate to have a client attend a party at the home of the therapist. It may be appropriate for the client to attend a retirement party, opening of a home office, or a particular social event, such as a rally to support the interests of science or a fundraiser for AIDS research. Hence, the reason for the party is very important. A party organized around a socially important topic may be more justifiable for a client and therapist to attend than a nonfocused event. It would never be appropriate for a client to attend a party at the home of the therapist without a focus for the event. In one case before the California State Board of Psychology, the therapist invited his patient to come to his home with her spouse for dinner. The therapist, who was also married, encouraged his patient and her spouse to join him in his hot tub, which later turned into a nude encounter. The dinner only involved four people, was casual in nature, and emphasized the social nature of the interaction. Later the therapeutic boundaries seemingly evaporated in the steam of the hot tub. This is an example of an inappropriate small party at the home of the therapist. Other parties for the purpose of socializing, laughing, drinking, or using illicit substances would never be appropriate for a client to attend, even though there may be numerous other people present, to say nothing of the problems therapists are getting themselves into by using illicit drugs or consuming alcohol excessively. Further, many therapeutic models prohibit all such contact.

The therapist should also determine the number of people attending the party. The more people at the party, the greater the chances that it may be appropriate for a client to attend. The fewer people at the event, the less appropriate it is for a client to attend. A party at the home of a mutual acquaintance in which 200 people are in attendance may not be a problem because the therapist may not even encounter the client during the event. Also, there would be no need for the therapist or the client to face the embarrassing moment of explaining how they know each other in such a large gathering. A small gathering is more intimate and creates a high probability that the subject of the client's and therapist's relationship will arise. Also, in a small gathering the conversation will be more personal and less superficial, leading to the potential for increased boundary blurring.

Timing is everything as well. A party or social gathering at night brings with it an aura of informality, while one during the day can be more closely associated with a legitimate business purpose.

One other factor must be considered: the nature of the client relationship. For purposes of this book, the term "client" is used broadly. Rules pertaining to clients who are in therapy with a provider must be interpreted more rigidly. But what about a case in which the clients are business entities, such as one would find in an industrial/organizational setting, or lawyers who have retained you to act as a consultant in a forensic case, or groups of therapists who are retaining you for the purposes of receiving training, or fellow board members, or students, psychological assistants, and employees? Would it not be the case that the rules should differ, depending upon the nature of the professional relationship? The model in university teaching involves continuous interactions between the faculty and the students inside and outside the classroom. From a personal standpoint, some of my most memorable learning experiences occurred while in graduate school, where there was a degree of talking, socializing, and being entertained at the home of one of my professors.

In summary, there is no absolute prohibition about attending a party with a client as long as the analytical model is used, an objective consultant concurs in the conduct, and the professional rationally concludes that there is minimal or no conflict of interest as well as no harm to the client. The answers to the above questions do not lead one to conclude that there is likely to be a problem with the activity, as the reader or the client would not actually or physically be transported to the party and the interests of the client are promoted in the activity. Consequently, it may be acceptable to attend a:

1. Wedding
2. Funeral
3. Baby shower
4. Retirement party
5. Award celebration
6. Election party
7. Open house at a business
8. Fundraising event at a home, such as for AIDS research, cancer funding, homeless advocacy, arts council, and so forth

Eating in the Office Together

I once encountered a case in which a lawsuit was filed against a social worker. The case involved a series of boundary violations, although there never was sexual contact between the therapist and the patient. Therapy began at an interval of once per week. There seemed to be a mutual attraction developing between the two of them. The patient entered treatment because he was obsessed with his ex-wife and he felt as though he was addicted to her. He could not stop fantasizing about her. After a few weeks, the therapist told the client that he should become addicted to her, the therapist, in order to forget his ex-wife. This message set the context for an increasing number of boundary violations. One of these involved eating lunch together in the office. During the first few weeks of the introduction of lunch into the sessions, the therapist offered several excuses: she was late, she was very hungry, she did not have time to eat, and she needed to eat to be alert during the sessions with her patients. She encouraged her client to bring in food so that he could eat with her as well. As time progressed, the therapist and client ate during every session together. The therapist allowed the client to purchase lunches for her. During several sessions the therapist asked the client, at the beginning of the session, to leave and find lunch for them to be brought back to the office. In addition, sessions were increased from once per week to several times per week. The therapist eventually began making sexually provocative comments to her male client.

In this example, lunch was a marking point in therapy. It was an initial departure from standard care constituting a minor boundary violation. It became the beginning of what is often referred to as the slippery slope; this is where one relatively minor boundary violation leads to a greater one, eventually leading to a serious breach of ethics. The process is not unlike the behavioral concept of successive approximation used in learning new behaviors. Each successive step leading toward the ultimate goal is reinforced and thereby adds to the individual's behavioral repertoire. In this case the social worker was sued and the case settled with a monetary payment to the client.

In deciding what to do about eating, the therapist must ask what the ultimate purpose is for the activity and how it promotes the interests of the client. A careful analysis must occur to ascertain whether eating lunch in the office with the client is the beginning of a slippery slope. As in our other discussions in this book, the theoretical orientation of therapists is relevant in that it may dictate certain rules and/or restrictions over and above the ethical and legal requirements of therapy. A psychoanalytic therapist must keep very strict boundaries as part of the theory for positive change in therapy (Gabbard & Lester, 1995). An analyst who eats lunch with a client is suspect because there is no room in the therapeutic model for this kind of boundary violation. However, a humanistic therapist or a pastoral counselor may find it is very appropriate to eat together. Likewise, a community psychologist or social worker may find it is a necessity to eat at a homeless shelter or a soup kitchen with patients.

Some community mental health centers have small restaurants where the seriously mentally ill at the center can eat along with their therapists. This is clearly not unethical but appropriate, humane, therapeutically productive, and socially beneficial. As previously mentioned, in Placer County, California, there is a kitchen/restaurant called Eleanor's Cupboard, which is sponsored by the Placer County Mental Health Department. Patients who suffer from serious mental disorders work at the kitchen and receive a salary. They often work alongside therapists employed by the mental health clinic. The therapists, patients, and other workers eat and work together. There are no questions regarding the motive for the activity and whose interest the kitchen serves. There may be those in more traditional psychotherapeutic schools of thought who would condemn such an endeavor. As Carl Sagan has said, "You can provide psychoanalysis to the schizophrenic or give him Thorazine" (Sagan, 1995); the implication is that science has offered better techniques for the treatment of those afflicted with mental disorders than theoretical methods.

Driving in a Car With a Patient

This is an activity in which there is no prohibition. The activity in no way places the situation in the prohibited class of the analytical model. Some therapeutic methods, such as systematic desensitization, support the therapist riding in a vehicle with a patient. Take the scenario of a 42-year-old African-American female who developed phobic symptoms pertaining to driving following a motor vehicle accident in which she was involved 2 years prior. The patient accidentally struck a 5-year-old boy, killing him instantly. The force of braking and the air bag deploying caused the patient to sustain soft tissue injuries. Ever since the accident she has been unable to drive without experiencing extreme anxiety. Whenever she drives down side streets in residential neighborhoods, she feels anxious and perspires, manifests heart palpitations, experiences elevations in heart rate, feels as though she is going to die, shakes uncontrollably, feels as though she actually hears her heart beating, and panics to such an extent that she pulls off the road.

A psychodynamic or psychoanalytic therapist might conduct talk therapy sessions in an office, designed to assist the patient in understanding the roots of her problem. In this instance it would not be appropriate for the psychodynamic therapist to drive in a car with a patient because the activity serves no therapeutic purpose and it is outside the theoretical boundaries of the clinician.

A behaviorist using cognitive-behavioral techniques, on the other hand, may begin by assisting the patient in changing her thoughts about driving, then teach relaxation techniques, possibly using hypnosis, followed by structured fantasies, to rate the anxiety reaction reported by the patient from 0 to 10, with 10 indicating severe anxiety. Some may even use biofeedback to measure the physiological reactions of the patient during a fantasy exercise. Once relaxation techniques are taught, the patient may be exposed to increasingly anxious images in order to test her ability to control the amount of anxiety she experiences at the time. This may lead to the patient and the therapist sitting in the automobile of the patient for the purpose of employing newly learned relaxation skills in an anxious environment. I recall an instance in which the therapy involved riding hospital elevators with phobic patients who were fearful of them. This successful technique led to patients who were symptom-free thereafter. It is conceivable that a therapist could actually ride in the vehicle of a patient to test the patient's ability to perform in vivo, although it may be wise to pay up all life insurance and disability policies prior to getting in the passenger seat with a client.

There have been numerous cases of inappropriate driving involving a client and a patient. In one case in which I was involved, the defendant, who was a therapist, worked with severely disturbed children in a residential center. On several occasions he took minors from the center on an outing and purchased liquor for them, then allowed them to consume it in his automobile. Later, he engaged in sexual conduct with some of them. Obviously, this example can be contrasted to the above in that the purpose of the activity in treating the phobic patient is exclusively directed at a legitimate therapeutic purpose, while the latter is not. The interests of the therapist in the first example are to assist the patient in alleviating her anxiety, while the latter case involves no motivation to assist the patient in reducing his patient's psychological problems. In fact, it is probable that the patient will be seriously harmed by the conduct.

There are cases where the therapist drives the patient around while discussing his or her problems. In these cases there is often no impropriety, although traditional therapists, from psychoanalytic or psychodynamic models, are appalled to learn of such conduct. But is it always unethical? Using the analytical model presented in this book, it is clearly not always unethical. The problem is that any professional who has boundary problems should work to prevent any departures from standard practice including riding in a car with a client. A simple drive around to view scenery and talk about issues of concern for the patient may be appropriate, provided the context has been made clear by the therapist. It may even be appropriate for a therapist to leave the office, view the new Lexus 400 of the patient, for example, or go for a short drive to demonstrate approval of the purchase to the client. As tempting as it may be, the therapist should not ask to borrow the car for the weekend. One psychiatrist who had treated adolescents for years funded by CHAMPUS would often drive his adolescent clients in his Mercedes to locations during his sessions with them. His practice of doing this is seemingly condoned by some psychiatrists reviewing CHAMPUS claims because the "patients may be helped." Although this may be unwise, it may not always be unethical.

What about a more ambiguous practice? What if the client feels more comfortable riding in a car and talking, feeling that this is the only place he or she can discuss difficult areas of life? I had a therapist friend, Dudley Hanchey (now deceased), who was a very experienced marriage, family, and child therapist. We lived far apart and would talk rather infrequently. Whenever he would sit in the passenger seat of my automobile, he would look over to me and say, "Now we can talk about personal issues." There would be no absolute prohibition against conducting therapy in a vehicle, although it is quite unconventional. The downside of this form of therapy is that it could be very expensive if an accident occurred. If your methodology allows for it, treatment planning is anticipated, and motives are pure, this form of therapy may be acceptable. For example, a therapist using systematic desensitization may ride in an automobile with a client as a means of therapy. As computer models develop with virtual reality programs, however, the need to actually ride in a vehicle with a client should diminish greatly.

Shopping With a Client

Upon seeing this in print, most rational therapists would probably think, "Why is this subject even being discussed?" Is shopping with a client always unethical? Currently there are no ethics provisions in any ethics code which prohibit a therapist from going shopping with a client. Of course, as an esteemed psychologist friend of mine often retorts, "There is no provision in the ethics code that states you shouldn't murder your patients, although everyone knows it is wrong to do so." The idea is that ethics codes are general documents designed to explicitly prohibit some behavior and set forth ideals for ethical therapists to follow in their practice. The analytical model used as an example in this book goes one step further. It sets forth a method of thinking about ethical problems that can be applied to every situation.

Going shopping may actually be appropriate in a case where the therapist and the patient are testing a new skill, such as assertiveness or relaxation therapy in what was previously an anxiety-provoking environment. Consider the case of *In the Matter of the Accusation Against Judith A. Johnston, PhD* (1995). In this case, during therapy, the psychologist took a significantly disturbed girl to various locations, including retail establishments. The patient was residing at a residential treatment center and the staff knew of Dr. Johnston's practice. During several of the outings, Dr. Johnston bought several items for her patient while they were shopping. The purchased items were insignificant in value and were not very expensive. The patient had no other significant support system in her life. In this case, and in applying the analytical model, the conduct did not appear to be unethical. The conduct was directed toward the best interests of the patient. It was not used as a vehicle to lead to some prurient goal of the therapist, but meant only to meet the needs of the patient. The shopping itself was under the auspices of a therapeutic session and not characterized as a social event.

Before therapy began, one initial aspect of this case involved very inappropriate and provocative clothing worn by the young client. The therapist concluded that this was detrimental to the adolescent and, therefore, convinced her to buy and wear more appropriate clothing. This activity in and of itself seemed to be of great therapeutic value for the patient, more so than sitting in a small room discussing feelings. This therapist did the right thing and sacrificed her own needs for those of the client. For that, she was prosecuted. Justice was eventually served in that she was exonerated.

Might it ever be appropriate for a therapist to take an indigent client to a clothing store to assist him or her in purchasing needed items such as clothes, pencils, paper, shoes, or a backpack? The answer is probably yes. The results of the analysis using the model would lead to a positive conclusion because the context is defined as appropriate and therapeutic, the appearance does not bring discredit upon the profession, and the motive of the therapist is pure and designed to further the client's legitimate needs. There would be no prohibition against future therapy because of the activity, nor was there any indication that the objectivity of either the therapist or the client was impaired. The free will of the therapist was in no way altered by the activity. However, arguably the free will of the client could be altered by the gifts and the experience of shopping. There was no indication in the facts of the case that the shopping created role confusion, probably because it occurred under the guise of therapy. The psychologist in question was psychologically stable, but the patient suffered from a number of significant psychological problems, creating the need for very carefully planned framing of the endeavor. In this case no objective consultant was used, although the use of one would have helped. An objective consultant could have concluded that the shopping excursions were not contraindicated. Finally, there was no evidence in the case that the conduct created a conflict of interest for either the therapist or the client. Incidentally, the psychologist was disciplined in this case mainly for her failure to keep records and for her report that she developed a long-term treatment plan but could not produce it upon request.

Shopping with a client to teach assertiveness skills may be appropriate. It is similar to the therapist who is treating a phobic patient and needs to obtain data about the patient in the environment where the problems arise. There are cases in which there is no legitimate therapeutic purpose for the shopping. In these cases the therapist usually initiates the activity as a means to be alone with a client with whom there is an attraction. The guise might be to assist the patient in buying a new car, help pick out a new dress or suit for an upcoming event, or window shop. The therapist is using this as a means to change the therapeutic relationship into a more personal one. There is usually one striking difference in cases where the therapist is using shopping to lure the client into more inappropriate contact: the lack of notes by the therapist. Therapists who are performing a legitimate therapeutic activity which would involve a departure from the office will record the event in detail in the patient's record. Those who are engaging in an out-of-office activity to promote their own improper needs will virtually never record the activity in the patient's record. In my experience concerning the review of numerous records involving therapist-patient sexual misconduct, I have been deafened by the silence of the record regarding what actually occurred between the therapist and the patient.

If the shopping has no legitimate therapeutic purpose, the client is too psychologically ill to understand the nature and meaning of the event, the therapist is pursuing his or her needs exclusively, and the objectivity of the therapist is diminished, we can assume a conflict of interest is present. This, in turn, may limit the free will of the patient and the therapist in future sessions and may make it less likely that the patient will return for treatment at a later date. Finally, the potential for harm is moderate with shopping, but it could easily lead to more harmful conduct as the therapist slips down the slope of bad judgment into the cavern of unethical behavior. Also, it is highly recommended to always consult with a colleague or a therapist prior to engaging in behavior that would be construed as being somewhat unconventional. Many times impartial consultants and therapists can detect the hidden motivations of the therapist which have remained outside the realm of introspection. There is no substitute for the use of a good objective consultant. Unfortunately, I have seen many cases in which an impaired therapist selected gutless consultants who were too afraid to share their own feelings and thoughts with that professional. It is critically important to obtain an opinion from an objective consultant or an experienced attorney who is aware of the laws, ethics, and cases regarding professional conduct. There are several very capable psychologist-attorneys who are currently in practice. These individuals can provide information and advice that will prevent harm to clients and keep the professional out of trouble. For guidelines on choosing qualified attorneys or consultants, see Appendices B and C (pp. 169-174).

Hot Tubbing With Clients

This portion of the book will provide a pleasant interlude to the complexities of the material previously presented. There have been a surprising number of cases where the therapist decided to spend time in a hot tub with a client. In some cases the therapist actually argued that hot tubbing with clients was for legitimate therapeutic purposes. Using the analytical model, it is virtually impossible to construct a situation where sitting in a hot tub with a client would not be a conflict of interest and/or would be ethical. Consider the case of *In the Matter of the Accusation Against Richard Boylon, PhD* (1994). Dr. Boylon treated numerous patients whom he claimed had been abducted by aliens. The abduction experience reportedly caused trauma similar to that of posttraumatic stress disorder. One of the treatment methods used by Dr. Boylon was to sit with his patients in a hot tub which was located in his backyard. The analytical model illustrates the numerous problems with this type of behavior. First, the activity occurred in the yard of the therapist, not in an office. Second, the appearance of the conduct to the public and the effect on the perception of the dignified nature of psychological practice was clearly tarnished. Third, the behavior itself had a tendency to create role confusion in the patients. Fourth, free will and objectivity of the patients and the therapists were seemingly impaired to one degree or another. Fifth, there was no evidence that the activity was discussed with an objective consultant, although there was evidence that other therapists knew of the conduct but failed to honor their duty and take steps to stop it. The clients who were treated to the hot tub experience were later diagnosed as suffering from Borderline Personality Disorder. They were not in a psychologically stable position to engage in any type of extratherapeutic contact with their therapist. In this case there was a clear conflict of interest. The clients needed long-term psychological help but they received an experience in a hot tub of little therapeutic value. In one case previously mentioned (*In the Matter of the Accusation Against Barbara Grimes*, 1997), the psychologist visited the home of the client, and they spent time in a hot tub together. As a result, the socialization eventually led to sexual activity. This is a case involving socialization that led to sexual misconduct and which would be viewed as being in the category of inappropriate conduct.

What about a situation where clients are treated at a comprehensive pain clinic especially for the treatment of chronic back pain? Would it be inappropriate for a therapist who is leading a group at the clinic to be in a hot tub with patients? Probably not, provided the context, motive, and objectivity were all clear and unimpaired. The clients and therapist must not be severely impaired, and the activity should be documented in a case record. Further, the activity and rationale behind it should be documented in the treatment plan. In the past 20 years, there has been no documentation in a patient's treatment plan for the need to participate in a hot tub experience with their therapist except in a formal pain clinic. The absence of the hot tub experience from the treatment plan is but one more piece of evidence leading one to conclude that most patient-therapist hot tub experiences are unethical breaches of therapeutic boundaries and are likely to cause harm to an already damaged patient.

Going to a Client's Home

Going to a client's home is another circumstance that may be ethical or unethical, depending upon the answers to the questions raised in the analytical model. An example would be:

> Dr. E. R. is treating B. L., a 26-year-old, very attractive female, who has clear borderline personality disorder features. Dr. E. R. is the seventh therapist to treat her in the past 5 years. B. L. has a very jealous boyfriend. B. L. plans to become a full-time model for a reputable agency in Los Angeles. However, years of prior abuse from her father have seriously hampered her confidence in herself. She is prone to periods of physical mutilation and threats of suicide, as well as acting out sexually. She has expressed her attraction to Dr. E. R. The doctor is also attracted to B. L. and on occasion has caught himself fantasizing about her.
>
> One night he receives an emergency page from B. L. She informs him that she is in love with him and that she will be forced to kill herself if they cannot be together. She demands that Dr. E. R. rush to her home immediately to attend to her. He does so without a witness or any type of help whatsoever. After he arrives at B. L.'s house, he learns that she also called her boyfriend. B. L.'s boyfriend arrives at the moment when Dr. E. R. is comforting B. L. in a long and passionate hug. The boyfriend becomes psychotically enraged and grabs a knife he brought with him. He slashes Dr. E. R. repeatedly while hitting him as well. Eventually the police arrive and the boyfriend is arrested.

This case presents interesting dynamics. On the one hand, the motive by Dr. E. R. was relatively pure: that of interceding in a patient's possible suicide attempt. Applying the model to this case leads to serious questions of the ethical nature of the conduct. First, Dr. E. R. was attracted to his patient, B. L. He was aware that she was attracted to him and that she was attempting to manipulate him into coming to her home immediately. Second, Dr. E. R. proceeded alone without fully assessing the probability that B. L. might actually attempt to kill herself. Third, Dr. E. R. was aware that B. L. had a very jealous boyfriend who might misinterpret his presence in her home. There are mixed motives; the doctor has some concern for the interests of the patient but is also proceeding to satisfy his own. The context of the situation was also ambiguous. On the one hand, he was going to B. L.'s home ostensibly to prevent her from killing herself. But he also seemed to be going to test the extent of their mutual attraction to each other. The appearance of the visit is problematic because Dr. E. R. went to the home alone. It is also likely that the objectivity of both Dr. E. R. and B. L. will be hindered by the encounter. In addition, Dr. E. R. did not consult an objective expert about what to do in the case. It is probable that no expert consultant would recommend to Dr. E. R. that he go to B. L.'s home at all under the circumstances, let alone by himself.

A clear conflict of interest arose in this scenario which had disastrous consequences for the doctor, the boyfriend, and the patient. Clearly the conduct was unethical in this instance. But are all visits to the home of a patient unethical? Absolutely not. As noted earlier in the discussion on attending parties, it may be appropriate under some circumstances to visit a patient's home. An example would be where your patient just completed a major work of art and is having a public showing at his or her home. Another example might be if, as a therapeutic task, one of your clients actually built a home or added a major addition to his home. A client could have taken up gardening as a stress management tool and requests you briefly view the project. These circumstances seem to fall in the direction of being appropriate supportive practice unless you are a strict psychoanalyst and/or psychodynamic therapist. Remember, the theoretical orientation of the therapist is relevant when the secondary relationship or conduct in question falls outside the prohibited class. If you do visit a patient's home, consider the following guidelines:

1. Never visit a patient's home alone. If there will be others present, then there is no need to bring someone with you. If no one else will be present, bring a friend, colleague, or witness to the location.
2. Only stay for a short period of time. An hour is considered a short period of time, whereas 2 hours is too long.
3. Keep the conversation superficial.
4. Be certain your motives are pure for the visit. Be able to articulate the therapeutic motives for your visit; they should be clear and logical.
5. Document the visit in the treatment notes of the patient, including the rationale for the visit.
6. If there is a moderate attraction to the patient, it is recommended that you not go to the patient's home at all.
7. Assess any potential dangers prior to going. If there are dangers, do not go.

8. Be suspicious of your own motives. In other words, is this the
kind of thing you have ever done before or never thought you
would do with a client?
9. Act formally during the visit.

Going to Sporting Events With Clients

Going to a sporting event with a client is another area where there
is controversy. In the movie *The Couch Trip*, Dan Ackroyd played an
antisocial personality disordered patient who was committed to an
Illinois psychiatric hospital and who had eventually escaped. He made
his way to Los Angeles and landed a job by mistake as a radio talk
show psychiatrist. In one scene he took a large number of his patients
in buses to a Los Angeles Dodgers baseball game. Incidentally, he also
sang the national anthem at the game and identified his patients who
were sitting in the bleachers. He asked for a round of applause for
them.

In this field, it is recognized that on occasion psychiatric hospital
staff will take their patients bowling or to other similar sporting events,
whether it be baseball, football, or basketball games. Although I am
inclined to conclude that the only legitimate sporting event trip would
be to view a baseball game, my own bias toward this sport should
never cloud my ethical analysis. It is understood and well known that
some psychiatric staff have been known to take their patients to a
skating rink, while others go to hockey games or tennis matches. In
some cases, the events are professional, such as an organized group
going to see the Chicago Cubs play baseball at Wrigley Field.

Taking patients on outings to sporting events has been recognized
as part of recreational therapy programs for over 30 years. Whether it
be to baseball, football, soccer, basketball, hockey, tennis, bowling, or
track events, the purpose is to provide a disturbed patient with a fun-
filled experience and for the patient to socialize, practice acting
appropriately in the real world, and observe others having fun and
controlling their impulses—although given the angry outbursts of some
fans and players recently noted in the news, including the infamous
basketball brawl in Detroit or the chair-throwing incident in Oakland,
the latter goal seems of dubious attainment. These events are planned,
are noted in the treatment plan of the patient, are documented in the
patient's records, and they usually occur with several chaperones and
with a more seriously disturbed population than is seen in most
individual therapy practices. The motives are pure for the therapists
who accompany the patients. There is no role confusion, because the
staff members act within their roles as care providers. There is no
detrimental effect on the perception of the profession by the general

public. There is no effect on the free will of either the clients or the therapists. The behavior is approved by supervising staff members. The context is clear in that the activity is a planned recreational function built into the treatment of the patients. The boundaries of the activity are very clear, and although the patients may be severely disturbed, the average mental health of the staff is quite normal. Hence, although it is arguably a multiple relationship to sit at a Cubs game at Wrigley Field, it is a perfectly ethical and appropriate adventure.

What about the case of an individual therapist who has two tickets to the San Francisco Forty-Niners game on a Sunday with seats located on the 50-yard line? He is aware that his next patient, a 29-year-old, very attractive single female, is an avid Forty-Niner fan. He has found himself very attracted to her to the extent that he has been fantasizing about her. Last night he contemplated asking his long-time psychologist friend who teaches ethics at a reputable university about the possibility of taking his patient to the game. He neglects to ask his psychologist friend about this problem. In his session with the patient he asks her to go to the game. She is ecstatic and agrees to go. He picks her up, goes to the game with her, and they both have a wonderful experience. They learn of their mutual obsession with football in general and of the San Francisco Forty-Niners team in particular. On the way home they stop at a bar called *Sports Heaven*. They have three drinks together and talk about the game. Later they go to the patient's house and begin hugging and kissing each other. Both voluntarily stop and prevent any further physical contact from occurring. It is discovered that the therapist does not document notes in the treatment plan.

This is a case in which the activity involved the use of therapy with a patient with the intent to find a date. This is to be contrasted from the planned sporting event where patients are taken to a game as part of a global recreational plan. The context in the preceding example was nontherapeutic. The motive of the therapist was not pure; that is, the activity was not directed toward promoting a therapeutic interest. There was direct avoidance of an objective opinion when the therapist could have consulted a colleague; in this case, the colleague would have undoubtedly advised against the activity. The experience at the game, that is, drinking and physical contact, all created confusion in the therapeutic relationship. The objectivity and free will of both the therapist and the patient were probably impaired by the events that occurred. In this case the therapist seems to indicate a level of psychological impairment that should have precluded him from following through with his plan. The patient was also vulnerable and particularly vulnerable to this type of scheme. Ultimately one could conclude that a significant conflict of interest was created by the activity.

The second example demonstrates how taking a client to a sporting event is inappropriate, while the first one shows how such an activity may be appropriate.

Art Openings

Attending art openings is a minor problem area. I raise this in this part of the book because it has arisen in several of my colleagues' practices. The scenario is usually that an artist/client is being treated in psychotherapy. One of the issues that arises in therapy is the creative difficulties the artist is facing—issues such as self-doubt, procrastination, fear of success, overcoming negative thoughts, and negative feelings which the client allows to prevent him or her from producing creative work. Issues described in this section apply to all of the arts: painting, music, dance, literature, poetry, sculpture, and so on.

Therapy focuses upon the blocks of the artist, generating motivation to work, challenging old and cumbersome thoughts that prevent the artist from creating. An example could be therapy that may even involve art itself in which the artist, a female, draws pictures to symbolize the conflicting feelings within herself. Eventually, therapy is successful in that the artist begins producing works that are of commercial quality. The artist is invited to participate in an art opening at a local gallery. She is proud of her work and of the psychological work you and she have accomplished together. Consequently, she invites you to the art opening. She writes a comment in the invitation that it is particularly important that you attend, given your valuable role in assisting and bringing her to this point in her career. Should you attend? If you do attend, what are the rules of your attendance? First, there is no prohibition against your attending such an event. To do so may place a burden on you to justify your conduct to a licensing board or ethics committee.

Reasons Not to Engage in Social Contact With a Client

1. Social contact may create confusion in the client.
2. Social contact may create confusion in the professional.
3. Social contact might lead to a slippery slope of ever-increasing boundary violations.
4. Social contact might harm the client.
5. Social contact might exploit the client.
6. Social contact might cause increased impairment in the client.

7. Social contact might create a lack of objectivity in the professional relationship.
8. Social contact might infect the professional relationship, making it less effective.

Rules for Social Interactions With a Client

Rule #1: It may be appropriate to have a social interaction with a client, depending upon circumstances.

Rule #2: Never have a social interaction with a client with a borderline personality disorder.

Rule #3: It is most likely considered unethical for teachers and supervisors to have lunch with their students and supervisees.

Rule #4: An example of an appropriate interaction may be lunch, conducted in the right social context.

Chapter 8

INSIDER TRADING AND USE OF OTHER INFORMATION GAINED IN THE COURSE OF PROVIDING PROFESSIONAL SERVICES

One way in which a professional may act contrary to the interests of a patient is when he or she uses information gained in the course of professional practice for personal gain. Not all such conduct is prohibited, but many types of behavior are clearly a conflict and are considered to be against the law. For example, imagine the delight you would feel to learn that a previously worthless parcel of real estate will soon become immensely valuable, as well as all of the nearby property; or that a corporation which is run by one of your patients is about to be purchased by a very large company at a value 10 times its current valuation in stock. Also, what if you discover from a patient that his or her corporation will have a special consultation opening for a therapist, at 10 hours per week at the rate of $125 per hour and that the position will be announced next Tuesday at 1:00 p.m.?

What if your patient is a general manager of the large new local car dealership and informs you that all their cars will be on sale for $500 under cost from the hours of 9:00 to 12:00 on Sunday for invited customers only? In addition, you learn that invited customers are those who have purchased two or more vehicles of a particular model in the past 5 years. You have never bought a vehicle from that dealership before but are told you can attend the sale. Also, suppose you know your patient has a Rolex watch worth $10,000 that he intends to sell by placing an advertisement in the newspaper to sell it for $3,000 in order to raise quick cash? What if your elderly patient owns a late-model luxury vehicle with only 18,000 actual miles on it and which is in perfect condition in every other capacity, and you learn that he plans to sell the car for $2,500 and will place it for sale in the next issue of the local newspaper?

Insider Trading

One major illegal activity by professionals illustrates this point. Insider trading of securities occurs when a person makes securities trades or passes information to another person for the illegal purchase of stocks or bonds, based upon inside information which is not accessible to the public. There must be an individual who is a source of information who is working for a company and obtains information that is, in effect, secret, and the receiver of the information acts upon the secret to make securities transactions. The most common scenario is when a corporate executive provides information to another person regarding a company which would likely affect the value of the company's stock. The receiver of the information then purchases stock in order to make money when the transaction occurs. This type of activity is referred to as insider trading, which is illegal.

There have been several cases of insider trading over the years. Consider the case of a therapist in California who had been practicing for more than 35 years. Therapist Mervyn Cooper of Santa Monica, California, was providing marital therapy to an executive of Lockheed Corp. Mr. Cooper was a licensed clinical social worker. The executive began seeing Mr. Cooper in 1994. During the course of therapy, the executive discussed an upcoming merger deal between Lockheed Corp. and Martin Marietta, two giant corporations in the defense industry. The value of the merger was $10 billion, and the Lockheed stock was expected to gain in value. The executive was one of only 30 people in the company who knew about the merger. Mr. Cooper arranged for a friend, who was a business executive, to place a very large order for the purchase of the stock. He bought more than $7,000 in call options of Lockheed Corp. When advised by the broker that the purchase was very risky, his friend told him that a news story relevant to the purchase would be announced by Lockheed Corp. very soon. As a side note, call options are considered to be one of the most risky investments available for investors. The nature of the risk itself and the amount involved raised immediate questions about the deal. The merger occurred on August 29, 1994, and Cooper earned approximately $175,000 in profit. Unfortunately, though, for Mr. Cooper, the Securities and Exchange Commission (SEC) watchdog unit, with sophisticated computer surveillance of possible suspicious trading, detected the large order. The outcome was that Mr. Cooper was caught and convicted. Initially, he faced a possible penalty of 10 years in prison and a $1 million fine, but the minimum sentence under current federal sentencing guidelines was 6 months.

Mr. Cooper pled guilty to felony fraud related to insider trading and agreed to return all profits and settle a civil SEC complaint against him for $110,000. The U.S. Attorney in the case said that Cooper destroyed patient records and provided false information to the SEC (*Los Angeles Times*, 1995). Later Mr. Cooper was subject to separate disciplinary action by the Board of Behavioral Sciences of California, the licensing board that regulates social workers. There was no evidence that the Lockheed executive intended to have Mr. Cooper use the information he shared in therapy for his own personal gain.

Imagine the sense of betrayal the executive must have felt when he discovered that confidential and highly sensitive information disclosed in therapy was compromised. In addition, the executive was most likely subjected to a criminal investigation to determine any complicity in the offense. The conduct of Mr. Cooper caused harm to his patient, the patient's wife, and the public. Disclosures such as this cause the general public to have less confidence in the sanctity and privacy of therapy. Unfortunately, the entire mental health profession can be discredited as a result of this type of case.

Consider the case of Dr. Robert Willis. Dr. Willis, age 52 at the time, was seeing Sandy Weill as a patient. Ms. Weill was the wife of the president of American Express Co. She was discussing the stress of her husband's business dealings, including his attempt to take over Bank of America. She told Dr. Willis that her husband was trying to persuade Shearson Loeb Rhoades to invest $1 billion in Bank of America. Dr. Willis told a friend of his about this information, and the friend purchased stock in Bank of America for Dr. Willis, himself, and two others. The Shearson investment deal was disclosed publicly thereafter, causing Bank of America's stock to rise. Dr. Willis and others made a total of $161,185.91 in profits. As a result of SEC suspicion, Dr. Willis and the others were caught by the SEC. Dr. Willis faced a maximum 10-year prison term and a fine of $500,000. He was eventually sentenced to 5 years probation, 600 hours of community service per year of probation, and a fine of $137,000. The U.S. District Court judge was reluctant not to send Willis to prison. His words should be heeded by all who are tempted to violate the trust of clients. Judge Caderbaum said:

> You violated your traditional duty of loyalty and sworn obligation to protect your patient's secrets. . . . I hope other physicians will be deterred from similarly betraying their patients' trust.

The judge further called Dr. Willis's conduct "reprehensible." She seemed to agonize about giving the psychiatrist probation given the nature of the conduct and the fact that Dr. Willis violated a therapy patient's right of privacy.

Many therapists become aware of corporate secrets in the normal course of providing professional services to clients. Clients who are corporate executives are often under high levels of stress, which affects their colleagues as well as their families. This can lead to marital problems requiring treatment. Consider the executive in a relatively new company. The executive is feeling great stress because for the first time his company is about to make a public offering of stock. He tells you that the stock may open at $10 per share but is probably worth $60 per share. If you place a buy order at the opening, you could make 600% profit. The multiple relationship component to all these incidents, which is a conflict of interest, is that the therapist would be using the client as an investment advisor and would be using confidential information obtained in the course of therapy to enrich the therapist in a way never intended as part of the therapy contract. Further, acting on the tip from a client betrays the trust of the client as well as the initial contract for treatment. The intended purpose of the client entering into a therapy fee agreement with the therapist was not entered into in order to provide stock tips for the therapist.

Therapists are often exposed to very sensitive information about publicly traded companies. This information could have a negative or positive impact in the stock price if it were disclosed. It is tempting for a therapist who is paid $80 per hour to try to earn money by making an investment that is most likely not speculative. The temptation is a normal feeling, while acting on it is a violation of law and ethics and is actually a felony. Both Borys (1992) and Koocher and Keith-Spiegel (1998) have discussed the ethical problems with becoming involved in a business relationship. There is an inherent violation of trust in a relationship that depends upon becoming involved in a business relationship. It is also bad for the profession as a whole, because when cases such as these are published, the public loses its trust and faith in the profession. The outcome may discourage potential patients from seeking therapy, especially those in real need of therapy. Besides constituting a violation of ethics, acting on an inside stock tip is a violation of the Federal Securities and Exchange Act of 1934. The SEC rule that applies is in Section 10(b-5):

> It shall be unlawful for any person, directly, or indirectly, by the use of any means or instrumentality of interstate commerce, or of the mails or of any facility of any national securities exchange,
>
> 1. to employ any device, scheme, or artifice to defraud,

2. to make any untrue statement of a material fact or to omit to state a material fact necessary in order to make the statements made, in light of the circumstances under which they were made, not misleading, or

3. to engage in any act, practice, or course of business which operates or would operate as a fraud or deceit upon any person in connection with the purchase or sale of any security.

The SEC rules prohibiting insider trading are generally applied quite broadly (see *Rochelle v. Marine Midland Grace Trust Co.*, 1976). This is an area in which the ethical breach also constitutes a felony. Hence, general proscriptions in ethics codes against breaking the law apply, as well as the specific provisions dealing with conflict of interest and dual relationships.

Real Estate Transactions

Another common area of gain for therapists from information obtained in therapy is in the real estate market. The most common scenario is where a realtor is in treatment and discusses a proposed zoning change that may lead to an increase in the value of a number of pieces of property in the area. In some cases, the therapist may be asked to invest in the purchase of property by the client. In other cases, the therapist may secretly try to buy land in the rezoned area without the knowledge of the client. Either way, the therapist is committing an act that is contrary to the best interests of the client.

In one case a therapist and a client bought a piece of property as an investment. They bought in an area that they both expected to appreciate dramatically. Unfortunately for them, the property values for the region dropped drastically, creating a situation where the mortgage was at a greater level than the value of the building. Thereafter the client decided to withdraw from the venture and asked that all of the initial investment, plus interest, be paid. The therapist, resistant at first, ultimately agreed in order to avoid litigation.

It is relatively easy to be discovered in these types of cases. So, for those therapists who are following Kohlberg's first level of moral development, the avoidance of punishment should drive them not to act on the tips received in therapy (Kohlberg, 1981). For others, the choice to refrain from doing so should be easy because it is the right thing to do. One of the ways in which cases are analyzed dealing with insider trading is whether the information acted upon could be obtained freely and easily through public access. If so, then there is no insider trading. This rule is probably not sufficiently strict for therapists. Real estate transactions generally involve a substantial amount of money. Because of this fact, the temptation to act on a tip by rationalizing the ability to do so is probably greater than in other circumstances. Situations such as zoning changes, unusual market trends, inside information on interest in a particular parcel of land, or highly motivated sellers based upon a sudden change in their personal finances give rise to the opportunity to gain monetarily. With the stakes so high, a professional must employ all of the resources available to do the right thing and refrain from acting upon the tip.

Tips on Business

A particularly difficult and complex area arises when a patient has a tip on a professional such as a physician, attorney, chiropractor, psychologist, or accountant, or a religious official such as a rabbi, minister, priest, or master. Patients will often recommend other types of professionals, including teachers, writers, nutritionists, physical therapists, and nurses. Many times the patient has been treated particularly well by a professional for a problem that also exists for the mental health professional treating that patient. Suppose the client had a serious herniation of a cervical disk. This caused constant pain, numbness, muscle tension, and radiated discomfort and weakness down the arm. The client sought treatment from a neurosurgeon and underwent a cervical disk operation that completely eliminated all physical symptoms. Suppose further that the mental health professional has the same condition. Is it unethical for the therapist to contact the neurosurgeon and seek consultation or surgery? The answer is, it depends. Neurosurgery is an area of medical practice with a limited number of practitioners unless one lives near a large metropolitan area or a teaching hospital. Even then, there are very small numbers of highly qualified practitioners. The best course in the previous circumstance is to find an alternative, which means finding a different doctor. If there are no other qualified individuals available, then the mental health professional must never disclose where he or she heard about the surgeon. In the era of managed care, this can be done relatively easily. In current managed care plans, referrals to specialists generally require a specific recommendation from a family physician charged with the primary care of the patient. It would be acceptable to mention to the primary care physician that a particular specialist had a very good reputation and that you wanted a direct referral. There cannot be a disclosure of the source of the information, because to do so would constitute a breach of confidentiality.

What about the case of a need for legal advice? Attorneys play an important role in our lives. In California there are approximately 165,000 practicing lawyers. There is no absence of attorneys in any locale in California. Hence, there would be no need to go to the same lawyer that a client is going to because other suitable alternatives exist. This is probably true regardless of the type of services needed, whether they be for estate planning, tort litigation, contract disputes, securities transactions, business law, business litigation, patent law, administrative law, maritime law, water law, health law, or criminal law. However, in Idaho there are only a small fraction of the attorneys that live and work in California. Attorneys often develop very close relationships with their clients, especially in a protracted case. A strong relationship may emerge that might compromise the primary or therapeutic relationship with another party. The problem is more difficult to deal with in rural areas and in states that are not so highly populated with lawyers and doctors. A complication to this problem is that often the best source for a referral to a doctor, lawyer, religious person, or other type of professional is a personal reference. However, the mental health professional must do whatever it takes to preserve the sanctity of the professional relationship with a client, even if that means sacrifice.

How about a referral to a religious person? Suppose the therapist is looking for a person to consult to deal with spiritual issues. The client happens to be a practicing member of the same denomination as is the therapist. The therapist has been unable to obtain the name of a religious leader in the area. The client discloses how valuable a particular person was to him. What if the denomination has a very small presence in the community? This increases the probability that a connection will be established between the therapist and the client, thereby violating the confidentiality and privacy of the client.

The problem can be more challenging when the therapist is in need of a support group run by volunteers, such as Alcoholics Anonymous or Narcotics Anonymous. If the therapist obtains a tip for a group from a client, and then attends the same group where the client is present, major ethical issues are raised as well as creating the possibility of infecting the therapeutic or other professional relationship. These situations have been referred to as "small world hazards" (Koocher & Keith-Spiegel, 1998). In a larger community there may be other sources of support. The problem is so significant that some professional groups have formed support groups for their profession. Lawyers have a group called "The Other Bar," which is specially designed for judges and lawyers who have problems with substance abuse.

Tips on Sales

Another set of problems can arise when the therapist learns of a special sale from a business during a session with a client. Consider the following example:

> May Cee is a 34-year-old client who is being treated for social skills deficits that are a by-product from her Bipolar Disorder. She works for a large retail store in the local area. During a session she informs you that there is going to be a special unannounced black rose sale on Friday evening from 8:00 p.m. to midnight. There are no formal announcements or advertisements for the sale in the media. You are in need of new clothes and you learn that clothing will be 50% off.

This is a dilemma. The facts as they are presented should cause a prudent and ethical practitioner to reflect before going to the sale. A few changes in the facts may lead to a different result, however. What if the sale is for automobiles and the cars will actually be sold for 10% under invoice and it is only announced for a few select customers? In the first example, it would most likely be ethical to go to the sale, while in the second scenario it would likely constitute a conflict. The analytical factors that are relevant include:

1. The likelihood of discovery, independent of the tip from the patient.
2. The amount of money involved; the greater the money involved, the more likely there is a conflict.
3. The extent to which going to the sale might expose the therapeutic relationship with the patient.
4. The effect that acting on the information might have on the therapeutic relationship. The greater the effect on the relationship, the greater the problem.

Gifts From Clients

Receiving gifts from clients has been referred to as a type of dual or multiple relationship, although it really defies logic to do so. It could easily present a significant conflict of interest, however. The rules on gifts have been fully addressed in a very thorough manner previously (Haas & Malouf, 2005; Koocher & Keith-Spiegel, 1998). The book by Haas and Malouf is particularly relevant as it pertains to gifts. The authors believe that the therapist should consider such things as the amount of the gift, the motive for the gift, the effect the gift will have on treatment, and the timing of the gift (Haas & Malouf, 2005). They conclude, "it is not unethical in all situations to accept a gift from a client" (p. 77).

I completely agree with the Haas and Malouf approach. A gift that is relatively inexpensive and given at a time when gifts are normally given, such as during a holiday, at the end of treatment, or for a special occasion done with no ulterior motive, is proper. It may even be proper for a therapist to give a small gift to a patient. Some situations involve gifts that ultimately play a role in contaminating the therapeutic relationship (*In re John Spurr, PhD*, 1997). Expensive gifts are inappropriate whether given by a client or a therapist. Further, making arrangements to have yourself actively involved in the will of a wealthy person, as was the case with one psychologist, is unethical and improper (*In the Matter of the Accusation Against Barry G. Bachelor*, 1997). In this case Dr. Bachelor surrendered his license to practice psychology which means he cannot practice in the state where he is licensed; the action is also reported nationally. As well as being unethical, it also may be illegal, in most states, to accept expensive gifts or be written into the will of a client. In addition, federal law states that any gift of significant value received by a professional must be claimed as income, according to IRS regulations.

Chapter 9

EMPLOYMENT OF CLIENTS

In the well-known and much publicized Menendez case, the brothers were treated in therapy by a psychologist named Dr. Jerome Oziel. Dr. Oziel also had a patient named Ms. Smith. At a certain point during therapy, a sexual relationship occurred between Dr. Oziel and Ms. Smith. Thereafter, Ms. Smith began working in the office of Dr. Oziel. Ms. Smith was working for Dr. Oziel at the time the sexual relationship was ongoing. Ms. Smith was asked to eavesdrop on a session Dr. Oziel was having with Erik and Lyle Menendez, wherein Erik was going to discuss his confession to the murders of his parents with Lyle. During the session, Smith overheard Lyle threaten to kill Dr. Oziel. At the end of the session, Lyle walked past Ms. Smith on the way to the elevator. Dr. Oziel believed that he, his family, and Smith were all in danger. He purchased shotguns for himself, his wife, and Smith. That evening he spent the night at Smith's home. The rest of the story is well known, in that the Menendez brothers were eventually convicted of the murder of their parents and the appellate case itself became a landmark case in the law of confidentiality (*Menendez v. Superior Court*, 1992). It also illustrates what can go wrong in an employment relationship where there are layers of relationships. Eventually, Dr. Oziel surrendered his license to practice psychology in the State of California.

Many problems can occur when a mental health professional hires a current or former client. Surprisingly, no professional organization has crafted a rule to preclude such post-service multiple relationships. If a current client is hired, numerous problems are created. The differential power relationship that exists between a therapist and a client is likely to become more pronounced. This may lead to greater inequities in the employment relationship. It may cause the client to be hesitant to raise important issues in therapy or may make the client reluctant to continue in treatment. If treatment has been terminated, the client may feel uncomfortable returning to therapy. Problems that led to treatment may eventually emerge in the employment relationship. The client may have work problems or even need to have time off because of an exacerbation of psychological symptoms. What happens if the client needs to file a worker's compensation case based upon work-related stress? The professional would be in the unenviable position of authorizing a claim against himself or herself. Oftentimes, work itself is considered to be a major source of stress in life. The client may feel very reluctant to raise work stressors in therapy in order to work on a long-term personality issue.

An additional problem is that of confidentiality. Employment of a client is a significant problem, given his or her access to sensitive information about other clients. The client may be exposed to client files, reports, medical information including HIV status, financial data, confidential telephone messages, reports about others from consulting professionals, and more. The financial information alone may include insurance policy numbers, assets and liabilities, debtors and creditors, credit card numbers, adverse credit report entries, checking and savings account numbers, or even records of bankruptcy. The client/employee may be called upon to type letters or reports with highly sensitive data about other clients. This may call for the person to actually retrieve and review the clinical files of others. With the advent of the Internet, sensitive and highly confidential background about a person could be transmitted to unauthorized individuals in seconds. The access to files could present other problems. What happens when a client reviews treatment of other patients with similar conditions? He or she may be upset that treatment is different and fail to understand why this is occurring. This could create additional problems in therapy that did not exist prior to beginning treatment.

The client may be unstable or may even be psychotic. Depending upon the severity of the client's psychological disturbance, the problems for the professional could be astronomical. Imagine a highly disturbed or even psychotic client answering the telephone or greeting clients. Not only is the situation unprofessional, but it is clearly taking advantage of the client who is vulnerable and subject to manipulation and abuse. Work is a particularly problematic place to mix clients. Most therapy is focused on clients' problems with work, family, relationships, and school. Work is a common source of stress for most people because it is a place where they spend 50% or more of their waking time. Hiring a current or former client is likely to confuse the situation at work and in therapy. On the other hand, there might be a situation where a client may benefit greatly by working for a therapist, particularly when the setting is in a public mental health center. Consider the case, previously discussed, of Eleanor's Cupboard, which is part of the program at Placer County Mental Health. Patients suffering from serious mental illnesses are employed at the kitchen, which is located next to the center office. The clients earn money and perform a wide range of duties, such as waiting on tables, taking orders, cleaning, and cooking, all done under close supervision. Efforts are made to ensure that no client receiving social security benefits earns more than the maximum allowable amount under the Social Security Administration rules. Clients receive extensive therapeutic benefit from this program. A strict application of the rules prohibiting multiple relationships would find such a program to be a violation of ethics. Such programs, however, provide essential therapeutic benefits to a population that is almost always underserved and one that has a high rate of unemployment. Working in an environment with support and praise, feeling as though one is making a contribution, and feeling needed are very strong therapeutic gains. No individual treatment, group treatment, or medicine, for that matter, will provide the same benefit. Centers have existed for years dealing with the developmentally disabled. Often these centers are called sheltered workshops. The success of such workshops is well documented.

On the other hand, Borys (1994) makes a compelling argument that therapeutic boundaries are curative for clients, per se. Borys indicates that there are elements within the boundary itself that make psychological healing, trust, and commitment to the process possible. Unclear from Borys' article is whether her analysis applies to structured work settings for the seriously mentally ill or those individuals with developmental disabilities. It may be that it only applies to mental health work performed in designated settings with a limited population. Koocher and Keith-Spiegel (1998) maintain that entering an employment relationship with a client creates problems of "power, control, and influence." They also note that an employment relationship with a client will create confusion in both the therapeutic and work environments.

For years attorneys have been struggling with the problem of involving themselves in business relations with clients. Such relationships have often been interpreted as creating an unfair advantage for the lawyer constituting unprofessional conduct (*Hunniecutt v. The State Bar of California*, 1988). In fact, the Hunniecutt case concluded: "Attorney's violation of fiduciary duty to a client is an act of moral turpitude warranting severe discipline" (p. 705).

Employment Concerns

Secretarial Staff

It has been determined that the most common form of employment of a client occurs in having the client perform some type of secretarial work. The client may answer the telephone, perform bookkeeping, greet other clients, file, or type reports, bills, letters, and other written work. He or she may write checks, manage a library, engage in practice marketing, or even schedule appointments. As in the *Menendez* case, many problems may arise. Often, the idea of performing secretarial work may arise while in therapy, when the client may inform the therapist that he or she is skilled in performing secretarial duties. The therapist may even rationalize and conclude that working in the office may be just the kind of therapy the client needs, as the therapist may, indeed, need secretarial assistance.

Often the client/employee is physically present in the office of the professional, the same office where therapy of the client/employee occurs. The client/employee not only sees the files of the other clients of the therapist, but may connect faces of clients with their files. In therapy practices, it is not unusual to have prominent people in the community call the office or be seen for services. The protection of their privacy is of paramount importance. Clients may have their privacy and confidentiality violated by the professional's employee who is also a client.

Issues that are generated at work pertaining to these contacts may make their way into therapy. This clouds the boundary of therapy and work. Further, the therapist may feel uncomfortable offering criticism to the client/employee at work, fearing this may exacerbate a psychological symptom. What if the issues for which the client/employee sought treatment had to do with unresolved conflicts between her and her authoritarian father? The client/employee acts out these conflicts at the office in an attempt to resolve them with her boss, who is also her therapist.

If the client/employee acts out her anger in a passive-aggressive manner, she could cause a great deal of damage to the professional and his or her clients. The actual tensions and conflict she experiences may increase in the situation and may result in acting-out behavior directed at the practice. What if the client/employee accidentally erases or deletes computer files? Will the therapist ever know if it was an accident or a passive-aggressive act? Probably not, although suspicions will run toward the latter motivation. Further, the client/employee may be reluctant to deal with these important work-related issues in therapy because her therapist is also her boss. The therapist may be uncomfortable making various interpretations or confronting the client/ employee or even providing psychotherapy to the client/employee. In this situation comes a restriction of behavior by both the client/employee and professional, which can only be detrimental to therapy as well as to the environment at work.

Many people with secretarial skills choose to work independently. Often, a typist will work at night at her or his home and enter into independent contracts with several professionals to type their work, ranging from letters to lengthy legal reports. The typist does not work out of the office of the professional but is separated from it. In some cases, materials to be typed are picked up outside the office, eliminating all direct contact with the confidential information of the professional. Regardless of the controls inserted by the professional, it is a bad idea to hire a current or former client.

In some cases a current or former client may be hired to perform limited work at an office. This limited work may involve performing reception duties, filing, or even assisting in the completion of managed care treatment reports. The professional working in a managed care environment faces much pressure. Very often, treatment reports may take 30 minutes to complete. If a therapist sees 30 patients per week and is conscientious about keeping good clinical records, a minimum of 30 hours will be used for direct services. The pressure to be able to complete the work often arises when the reports and paperwork must be completed. Returning telephone calls may take another 2 to 3 hours. That may leave little time for professional reading, attending workshops, or specialized research to learn better methods of providing services to clients. Few secretarial personnel have expertise in dealing with the secretarial or business demands of a managed care company. A professional who locates an individual expert in the area may want to hire that person immediately. If the person is a current or former client, therein lies the dilemma. The problems with such an act are the same as those mentioned previously. Even if the employee is hired on a limited basis, the rules against multiple relationships would prohibit the hiring (APA, 2002, § 3.05; American Psychiatric Association, 2001, § 1.1; AAMFT, 2001, § 1.3; ACA, 2005, § A.5.d.; NASW, 1999, § 106(c); AAPC, 1994, § III). The employee would have access to highly sensitive information about other clients. In addition, there would still be, at least theoretically, a differential level of power in the relationship created by the therapist-patient relationship. There is an unequal balance of power in an employer-employee relationship. It becomes more unequal when the therapist-patient template is placed on top of it. Further, the hiring may create hesitancy on the part of the former client to return to the therapist for future services.

Bookkeeping Services

I chose to list bookkeeping services separately because they are often performed by a person who functions as an independent contractor. It is not unusual for a bookkeeper to have several clients and obtain contracts with several individuals. Many bookkeepers work from a home office. Hence, this is a different situation from having a client/employee come into the professional office to perform services. Despite the differences, the same basic problems of actual or potential conflict remain (Borys, 1992). In addition, a bookkeeper is generally not exposed to clients' clinical records. However, the contract employee must have access to a client's diagnosis, frequency of treatment, insurance carrier information, number of prior sessions, and, in some instances, credit information, such as a credit card or a checking account number. The client would also have access to detailed data about the professional's financial status, including the amount of money the professional makes each week. This fact alone could create problems, given the differential in pay between what bookkeepers and mental health professionals earn. A bookkeeper who is struggling to pay his or her financial obligations making $15 per hour could easily become resentful of a social worker or a psychologist earning $90 per hour. The issue is likely to be more abstract for a bookkeeper seeking treatment who is not recording specific data from her or his therapist's practice.

As in other employment relationships, there is the possibility that problems will arise. What if the bookkeeper makes serious errors resulting in loss of revenue for the professional? Or even worse, what if the errors cause the Internal Revenue Service to look closely at the professional's business? What happens when there is conflict between the therapist and the client/bookkeeper? The client may believe the therapist has an unfair advantage in a verbal argument or that he or she is using information gained in the course of treatment against the client. The client may feel that the advantage of the therapist is so great that direct response will be unsuccessful. This may lead to passive-aggressive behavior. The last thing a mental health professional wants or needs is a passive-aggressive bookkeeper working in his or her office. Most importantly, the risk is high that the multiple relationship will be detrimental to the client/bookkeeper. The APA (2002, Standard 3.04) ethical code lists one of the most important standards to always keep in mind: Avoid Harm. Consider the words of Hippocrates (Edelstein, 1943) in light of this scenario:

> I will follow that system or regimen which, according to my ability and judgment, I consider for the benefit of my patients, and abstain from whatever is deleterious and mischievous.

The harm that may occur is that a client/employee who is in need of care may feel unable to pursue it with the professional who hired him or her, and may be untrusting of others because of the experience with the therapist/employer. Like the Hippocratic oath that has reminded physicians of their solemn duties for over 2,000 years, there is need for mental health professionals to take and follow an oath as well.

Babysitting

There have been several cases where a mental health professional has employed a client to perform work as a babysitter at the home of the therapist. Consider this scenario:

> Dr. Buz E. Bee is a very busy marriage and family therapist. He begins treating a 15-year-old girl who has been depressed for years. The girl lives with her aunt since she was removed from her home because she was abused by her father. She has no independent source of income and needs a job. Buz is married and has three children. He and his wife, Mrs. Bee, are invited to attend a dinner meeting of the local marriage and family therapists association. Dr. Bee is scheduled to receive an award for significant contributions in the field. Buz trusts his 15-year-old patient and also feels sorry for her. At the last minute the regular babysitter for the Bees cancels because she is sick. Dr. Bee has no other alternatives, so he contacts his patient. He offers her $6.00 per hour to come over to his house to babysit. He picks her up and takes her to the home where she watches the Bee children for 5 hours without incident. The next day, Buz sees his patient in therapy. The first comment by the patient is, "Doctor, you have wonderful children and a great house."

This happens more often than one would like to think, especially in a rural environment where there are limited resources for therapists and babysitters. Although there is no express prohibition against hiring a client as a babysitter, the possible problems noted earlier in employing a secretary are present along with some additional ones. The babysitter has access to the home of the therapist. There may be many confidential documents and items in the home. It is not unusual for a babysitter to look through the house for interesting materials, objects, documents, and other things belonging to the party hiring him or her. The therapeutic boundaries are clearly violated and blurred by the different relationships that exist. What if the babysitter is very angry at the therapist for a confrontation that occurred in a session? The babysitter may discover bruises on the children and make a report to Child Protective Services. Another possibility is that the babysitter may hurt the children emotionally or physically. Taking action as one would with a babysitter by either firing or reporting the babysitter to the police or protective services would clearly have an adverse effect on future therapy.

Might there ever be a time when it would be ethical to hire a client to be a babysitter? There are probably some rare circumstances when it may be acceptable to do so, if all of the following apply:

1. The client is not suffering from any type of serious mental disorder.
2. The client has a mild adjustment disorder.
3. Treatment is short term only and has ended.
4. The therapist is psychologically healthy.
5. The therapist and client live in a rural area.
6. The guardian of the client is consulted.
7. The payment for services in each setting is separate.
8. There is some type of necessity.
9. No other resources exist, or the client has a legitimate need for money.
10. The activity of hiring a client to be a babysitter is not prohibited by law.
11. The theoretical orientation of the therapist does not prohibit such conduct. An example of this would be if the therapist is a psychoanalyst. There is no justification for this conduct in the analytic model. (Some have tried to take this theoretical orientation argument to an extreme level. They have argued, for example, that humanistic therapists have a different standard of care as it pertains to sexual conduct with a current or former patient.)
12. The parent of the babysitter, if he or she is a minor, approves of the conduct.

It is not a good idea for a therapist to hire a client to be a babysitter. However, there is no law or rule that prohibits this activity. The ethics codes are written more generally with specific prohibitions in sexual conduct. There is no antibabysitting clause. There are a few lawsuits alleging a breach of the standard of care for allowing a client to babysit. None of these lawsuits cited babysitting as the sole violation of appropriate professional practice.

House Cleaning

A type of dual relationship often entered into with a client by a therapist is that of employing a client to clean the therapist's home. The most likely scenario is as follows:

Ti Dee is a client in treatment to control obsessive-compulsive behavior. She is so compulsive that she cleans her house twice per day and her bathrooms every night. Every picture in her house is perfectly straight and every towel and piece of clothing in the home is folded neatly and in its designated place. At the therapist's advice Ti opens a house cleaning business. The therapist, Ima Mess, PhD, is in desperate need of a house cleaner since she has a very busy practice and does not have time to clean. After Ima notices Ti straightening up the waiting room, she asks Ti if she has any openings. Ti agrees and begins cleaning Ima's home every week for a fee of $50.

This is not an uncommon scenario. The same problems noted above for babysitters and generally for hiring clients apply to this situation. Additional problems may exist. As a result of this scenario, the client has complete and unrestricted access to the home of the therapist. This means the client could easily view highly confidential and private information about the therapist or his or her patients. If, as is the case in most professional homes in 2006, there is a computer, the client could access confidential files. Also, the idealized sense of the therapist which causes the client to have faith in the process and success of therapy may be shattered by the discovery of private possessions of the therapist. Further, the client may begin to realize what great differences exist between the sloppy, somewhat physically unkempt therapist and the obsessively neat client. This may lead to discomfort in therapy as well as a lack of confidence in the therapeutic process.

The matter could be more complicated if there is an offset of charges for therapy based upon the cleaning work completed. Regardless, the therapeutic boundaries are blurred when the professional hires the cleaner. There is always the risk that something discovered by the cleaner may make him or her less comfortable raising certain issues in therapy. Another problem that may occur is when the therapist has blurred other boundaries with other clients. If this is public knowledge, the client, who is a cleaner, may be offended when the therapist tries to set limits with him or her.

Repair Personnel and Cleaners

Another complicated area is in dealing with repair personnel. In the increasingly specialized world of repairs, it is not unusual to need the services of workers with expertise in plumbing, electrical repairs, carpentry, lawns, heating and cooling, dishwashers, washers and dryers, burglar alarms, fireplaces, computer repair, automobile repairs, and garage doors. Today it is probably easier to find a lawyer or a doctor than it would be to find an electrician or a plumber. The biggest problem occurs when the mental health professional is treating a person who has special skills and the professional has a need for the client's services. Suppose that you are treating a person who turns out to be the best plumber in the city where you work. This person has a stellar reputation for producing high quality work and has reasonable fees. You suddenly develop a major leak in your home toilet requiring immediate attention. Do you call your client to assist you or even to ask for a referral? What is the conflict in making contact with your client? Suppose you do call your client and he comes to your home in the evening. He discovers that your bathroom is extremely dirty with mildew, sinks that have not been cleaned for months, and a toilet that is both leaking and plugged. He might begin to question the quality of services you could provide to him because of living in conditions such as this. This alone could be damaging, because an important component of the success of treatment is the patient's belief and trust in the therapist.

Another circumstance that arises between a client and a professional is when the client owns and operates a carpet cleaning business. This is the kind of business that is fraught with financial risks for the cleaners and material risks to the expensive carpet of the person having his or her office or home cleaned. Over the years there have been numerous scandals involving carpet cleaners. The business relationship is one of independent contractors. Carpets in both the home and the office need to be cleaned. If the professional hires the client to provide cleaning for the office, at some level, the client will be happy because he or she will gain business. There is somewhat of an expectation in the business world that business owners who know each other will transact business in each other's stores. Hence, the carpet cleaner/client will be expecting the social worker or psychologist to use his or her services for cleaning.

If the professional agrees, the cleaner obtains access to the home and office. The chances of accidentally encountering confidential material or information that would be detrimental to the primary therapeutic relationship is quite high. What if the cleaner picks up a telephone bill on the therapist's carpet? Suppose the bill contains a large number of 1-900 (sex conversation telephone lines) calls that are 45 minutes in length each. The client may be so disturbed by the discovery that future therapy is impossible, because the belief and trust in the inherent goodness and effectiveness of the therapist may be destroyed. The cleaner could find less emotionally charged but also potentially disturbing material, such as dirty clothes on the floor, dog excrement on the carpet, books and papers scattered all over the home and office, computer disks out of their cases, compact disks lying on the floor, crayon marks on the walls, or other evidence of a messy lifestyle. The problem is that the secondary relationship (carpet cleaner-consumer) may interfere significantly with the primary relationship (therapist-client).

Problems may arise in all secondary business relationships. The likely scenario is when the therapist is unhappy with the work of the client. Suppose in the process of cleaning the house the carpet cleaner burns several holes in the $5,000 Persian rug in the living room. The therapist may protest vigorously and decline to pay for the costs of the cleaning while demanding full compensation for the loss of the carpet. The cleaner may deny he or she was the cause of the burns, refuse to pay, and/or blame the therapist for leaving such an expensive rug out in the rooms that were to be cleaned. It is virtually impossible to keep the conflict out of the therapeutic relationship, resulting in a piercing of the boundaries (Borys, 1992, 1994). That is, the conflict surrounding the cleaning will affect what occurs in therapy, and vice versa.

Mowing Lawns, Gardening, and Yard Work

A common demand of any homeowner is to keep up with the required yard work. Mowing one's lawn, pulling weeds, trimming trees and shrubs, planting flowers and trees, growing vegetables, fertilizing a lawn, raking leaves, and cleaning up debris that has blown into the yard are tasks that some people love, while others, including myself, become physically sick at the prospect of engaging in such work. Like many areas of modern life, there are specialists who are experts at performing all of the duties and chores required by one's yard. In addition, many teenagers earn money doing yard work during the summer months. The fees usually involve a standard hourly rate common to the community; Hollywood versus Murphysboro, Illinois. Suppose your client owns a gardening and lawn business and you have a desperate need for yard work to be completed by someone competent. Is it always unethical to enter into an arrangement whereby you contract separately to have your client mow your lawn while you provide services to him or her? Most ethics writers would probably conclude that because it is a multiple relationship, it must be unethical.

The answer to this circumstance is not quite as easy as that given for the secretarial work. The problem could be further complicated in a rural environment where there are few therapists and one gardener. One case that is very illustrative of the problem and of bad judgment involved a psychologist, Dr. Oziel, who provided therapy for a patient. The patient could not afford the cost of psychological services, so he entered into an arrangement whereby the patient would perform construction-type work on the home of the psychologist in exchange for therapy fees and costs. The patient removed trees from the psychologist's yard, performed carpentry work at the home of the therapist, installed a sprinkler system, demolished a retaining wall, and engaged in landscaping at the home of the psychologist. The arrangement became problematic in that the cost of therapy ended up being more than a thousand dollars per hour when the calculations were computed for the time the client spent on the psychologist's home versus the therapy provided to him. The client complained to the California Board of Psychology (*In the Matter of the Accusation Against Leon Jerome Oziel, PhD*, 1986). Dr. Oziel received probation and was subsequently involved in the Menendez murder case which led to his license revocation. It appears the psychologist did not learn from his prior disciplinary action.

Borrowing Money From or Investing With Clients

Situations where a therapist or provider of health care borrows money from a client are not that uncommon. In addition, there are numerous cases in which a client and a therapist invested in various projects together. Consider this scenario:

> T. Cher is on the faculty at the University of Calivada. He is active as a professor in that he teaches two classes, one in psychopathology and the other is in supervised practicum. His research interests include group therapy. He runs a group for students that is modeled after the growth groups of the late 60s and the early 70s. There is a graduate student in the group, Bill Unaire, whose parents own a large disk operating factory for computers. T's salary is not very high and he needs money to pay for his brand new computer system. After group one day, Bill approaches T and asks him why he seems down. T explains that he needs a new home computer system for his research and writing. Bill says, "I have lots of money and I'd like to help. T accepts the check for $10,500. Bill continues to attend group but starts to become uneasy a year later when no payments have been made to him.

Circumstances like these actually occur. Often the reason the therapist needs money is a good one. The therapist, however, is using his or her unequal power balance to get the client to say yes and provide money to him or her. This creates a debtor-creditor relationship for the client and the therapist. As previously discussed with regard to students and supervisees, no matter how much money the client has or how well-intentioned the offer to loan money to the therapist is, the acceptance of money from a client is a prescription for disaster.

In one case a therapist, along with partners, borrowed approximately $40,000 from a wealthy client for a business venture. The loan was legitimate and included a contract with repayment terms. The partners were supposed to share the risk equally and make payments to the client. The partners defaulted on the loan, leaving the psychologist left to pay the entire balance by herself. She made payments for a while but could no longer do so. The client became angry and filed a licensing complaint. The case was heard before an administrative law judge and the psychologist's license was revoked, although the revocation action was stayed and 5 years probation was ordered.

In yet another case a mental health professional was providing treatment to a patient later diagnosed as suffering from a borderline personality disorder. Therapy progressed and the professional believed the patient was much healthier than when she began treatment. The patient found a condominium to purchase but needed extra money. The therapist decided, at the request of the patient, to invest in the condominium with her. He was convinced that the property values were stable, at a minimum, and that they were likely to grow in value in the future. The patient actually resided in the condo. A few years later the property values in the area plunged, making the value of the condo much less than the amount owed on the property. The patient wanted to move out and asked the therapist to buy her portion of the condo at the original valuation. When the professional refused, the patient threatened a lawsuit and a complaint to the licensing board. The professional opted to pay the client and sustained a loss of thousands of dollars as a measure of risk management.

The problem arises at the beginning of the transaction. The question is whether the influential position of the therapist can in any way be minimized to give the client informed and free choice. Informed consent in all matters in a professional relationship is required for mental health professionals (Ebert, 1997). One form of borrowing is to have a patient invest in the practice/business of the professional for a designated return on the investment. The client is in the same role as a bank, credit union, savings and loan, or the Small Business Administration. The money comes directly from the client into the accounts of the professional for use in a part of the business, whether it is to purchase equipment, buy property, or meet a payroll. The client becomes a partner in the business, leaving three different levels of a relationship in existence: client-therapist; debtor-creditor; and business partner-partner. The more levels of relationship added to the primary treatment relationship, the more likely it is that complications, confusion, and, ultimately, harm will be heaped on the client.

Lending Money to a Client

One problem area rarely discussed is the reverse of the above. Sometimes mental health professionals loan money to clients. There are a number of circumstances where this occurs. Are all of these bad?

The answer is probably not. Consider the following scenario adapted from an actual case:

> Al Truist is a therapist who treats children between the ages of 6 and 12. Most of the children are separated from their families and are in the government child protection system. Some are in group homes, others in temporary shelters, while others are in foster placement with a few in residential treatment centers. Al begins treating Heather, an 8-year-old female who has been abandoned by her family. There is evidence of significant early deprivation, including minimal love given to her between the ages of birth and 2 years, neglect in feeding and clothing, and possible physical abuse. Al sees Heather once per week at the treatment center. He often takes Heather on outings into the local community. Heather does not have sufficient money to have decent clothes to wear. Al decides to loan Heather money so she can buy a few pants, a dress, and several tops, including a sweatshirt. The loan is offered without any requirement that Heather reciprocate in any way other than by paying it back eventually.

The loan in this instance is a truly altruistic act by the therapist. Is it wrong? Suppose Al was a psychoanalytic therapist. Would that affect the analysis in any way? There is no prohibition in any ethics code against loaning or giving money to a client. There are relevant provisions in the codes to consider, however. For example, if the loan was made at an interest rate detrimental to the client, the dual relationship and avoiding harm provisions of each code would be violated (APA, 2002, Sections 3.04, 3.05, and 3.06; AAMFT, 2001, § 1.3; NASW, 1999, § 1.06(c); American Psychiatric Association, 2001, § 1.1; ACA, 2005, § A.5.d.; AAPC, 1994, § III). This would constitute a significant blurring of boundaries that would cause harm to the client and therefore be unethical (Borys, 1994). The therapist might employ some of the well-documented rationalizations to justify both the loan and the interest rate (Pope & Vasquez, 1991, 2001). But what if there was no interest rate, or there was no definitive timeline for repayment; that is, the act was truly altruistic? Using the analytical model, that loan may be ethical. It would create a multiple relationship, but not one in the prohibited class. The analytical factors would not lead to a direct conclusion that the conduct was improper. Mental health professionals should never hide behind the prohibitions of dual relationships to withhold concrete help, even if it is for money, food, clothing, or shelter.

Changing the facts in this scenario can totally alter the ethical conclusion. Suppose that Heather is a 31-year-old adult. She needs money desperately for her business. Al loans her several thousand dollars at a 20% interest rate with payments beginning immediately.

There is no altruism in this set of facts. There is, however, exploitation of the client. It may be that the client would never agree to accept money with such a high interest rate but for the existence of the therapeutic relationship. Ultimately, the better solution may be to give money to an institution that might assist a client; in other words, add a legitimate third party to the equation. But the truly altruistic loan or gift may not be unethical, per se. The most important distinction in the two examples is in the motivation for the act. In the first act, Al is motivated by his desire to genuinely assist another human being without benefit for himself. This pure act of kindness is motivated by a higher principle of virtue coming from within a character structure that is advanced and healthy. The latter act is motivated by a desire by Al to gain financially at the expense of the client. There is no duty or virtue in his actions in this example. To the contrary, his act reflects a stain in his character. He has allowed greed to overcome his professional judgment.

There may be circumstances where it is ethical and appropriate to loan money to a client rather than give it to him or her as a gift. For example, the client may need $10 for cab fare to return home or $7 for a meal because he or she has not eaten for a day, or $20 to buy a jacket during cold weather. In such cases, the following rules should apply to loans to clients:

1. The loan must be necessary to meet an immediate need (e.g., cab fare).
2. No interest may be charged for the loan.
3. The loan amount should be small (e.g., less than $50).
4. There must be a short period of time for repayment, preferably within 1 week.
5. There must be no ulterior motive on the part of the therapist to loan money to the client.
6. There must be no obvious ulterior motive identified in or by the client to take the loan.
7. The therapist must be certain the loan will not be used to purchase substances such as alcohol or drugs.
8. The therapist must be prepared to turn the loan into a gift.
9. The loan issue should not interfere with therapy of the client.
10. Preferably, the loan terms should be documented and signed by the client.
11. Other resources for the client must be unavailable or impractical.
12. The therapist is psychologically healthy enough to deal with the boundary issue created by the loan.

13. The therapist's independent consultant has generally approved of the arrangement.
14. Under the totality of the circumstances, the loan is appropriate and ethical.

The professional should be aware that a multiple relationship is being created by the loan. But not all such relationships are unethical, exploitative, or harmful to the client. It is the multiple relationships that either do cause or are likely to cause harm to a client or those that violate a fundamental right involving the client that are unethical.

Reasons Why It Might Be Acceptable to Hire a Client

1. Genuine need for the client's services.
2. Lack of alternatives in the community.
3. Trust in the integrity of the client based upon knowledge gained in treatment.
4. Nature of the professional contact was very limited, thereby deceasing the probability of conflict.

In summary, the following rules should be considered.

Rules Regarding Hiring a Client

Rule #1: Do not hire a client as an employee.
- Do not hire a client to be a secretary.
- Do not hire a client to be a babysitter.
- Do not hire a client to clean your house.
- Do not use a client to perform repair services.
- Do not ask your client for recommendations for experts in a field unless it is the last alternative.

Rule #2: Do not hire a client as an independent contractor.

Rule #3: Do not hire a former client as an employee.

Rule #4: There are only a few exceptions to the rules.

Rule #5: Do not borrow money from a client.

Rule #6: Do not lend money to a client except in an unusual situation and if it is a small amount.

Chapter 10

WORKING COUPLES

Today it is common for married or other committed couples to be employed. It is not unusual for married couples or partners to be professionals. There are many types of professional couples, including the following combinations:

1. Physician-Physician
2. Psychiatrist-Marriage and Family Therapist
3. Psychiatrist-Attorney
4. Psychiatrist-Psychologist
5. Psychologist-Marriage and Family Therapist
6. Attorney-Marriage, Family, and Child Counselor
7. Attorney-Psychologist
8. Social Worker-Social Worker
9. Psychologist-Psychologist
10. Psychologist-Business Person
11. Pastoral Counselor-Physician
12. Counselor-Chiropractor

There are many other combinations, but the preceding examples are a representative sample of professional couples. It is not unusual for a couple to be mental health professionals in practice together. Some couples have engaged in marital and family therapy together as a team. Others work in the same office and cross refer, particularly if each is specialized in a different area of mental health practice.

Few, if any, have written about the ethical conflicts created by couples who are working professionals. It is particularly problematic for mental health professionals and attorneys because there are strict rules of confidentiality that preclude disclosure of information about clients to anyone, especially a spouse, except under limited circumstances (APA, 2002, Standard 4; NASW, 1999, Standard 1.07; AAMFT, 2001, Principle II; ACA, 2005, Section B; AAPC, 1994, Principle IV; American Psychiatric Association, 2001, Section 4). The problem is not particularly difficult to deal with in a large community where there are numerous resources available for consultation, medical care, legal assistance, and other professional services. It is much more complicated in a smaller community or in a special community, such as in a church organization or in the gay and lesbian community, where there is an expectation that a multitude of resources will be made available from within the social entity. There are also problems when there are scarce resources in a larger community. Such is often the case for psychiatrists, certain medical specialists, such as neurosurgeons or pediatric neurologists, or mental health law attorneys. Consider the following example:

> Sigh Chiatrist is a physician who is board certified in psychiatry. He works in a city with a population of 25,000. He is one of three psychiatrists in the city and the only one most agree is competent. His wife, Mary G. Counselor, is a marriage and family therapist working in a different office. She often has clients who are in need of medication management. After several frustrating attempts at trying to find a psychiatrist or a family practice physician to provide medication support for her clients, she finds that it is in the best interests of the client to refer them to her husband, Sigh. She does so, but prior to making the referral, she discusses the situation with her client, engages in full disclosure, and gives three other names of psychiatrists in the next city for the client to choose.

This is a clear case of a potential conflict of interest, and it is certainly a multiple relationship. However, it may not be an unethical act or a relationship that is unlawful or unethical. Strict psychoanalytic therapists may have serious doubts about the appropriateness of such conduct. They consider what is in the best interests of the client. Full disclosure, as well as keeping the client's interest as a priority, may allow for some unusual relationships that, initially, may seem inappropriate. What if the facts are changed somewhat in the hypothetical? Suppose that Mary G. will often refer her clients to her husband, who is an attorney, for legal work. She does not disclose the relationship. The community has numerous other attorneys who are very competent. With this change of facts, the ethical problem is clearer in that there is no disclosure, the rules on informed consent have been violated, there are adequate alternatives available for the client, and there are many referrals that ultimately result in financial gain for

Mary G., based upon the number of clients being referred. This would be a circumstance that would present significant ethical problems. A definitive, all-encompassing rule on the subject would be virtually impossible to fashion and would probably not be in the ultimate interests of patients. There is no current prohibition in any mental health professions ethics code against referring a patient to a family member provided there is no special financial remuneration for the referral.

There are several relevant provisions of ethics codes that provide guidance. One such provision that appears either explicitly (APA, 2002; Edelstein, 1943) or implicitly (American Psychiatric Association, 2001; AAMFT, 2001; NASW, 1999; ACA, 2005; AAPC, 1994) is the rule requiring professionals to avoid harming their patients. The American Psychological Association rule is very clear and unambiguous. It provides at Standard 3.04: "Psychologists take reasonable steps to avoid harming their clients/patients, students, supervisees, research participants, organizational clients, and others with whom they work, and to minimize harm where it is foreseeable and unavoidable." Also consider AAMFT Standard 1.3: "Marriage and family therapists are aware of their influential position with respect to clients, and they avoid exploiting the trust and dependency of such persons."

In addition, rules about confidentiality, informed consent, competence, and exploitation, which appear in all mental health professions' ethics codes, provide general guidance in circumstances not specifically denoted or even anticipated in the code. The rules regarding informed consent are particularly important because modern mental health practice requires a professional to carefully inform clients of numerous aspects of mental health service (Ebert, 1997). Informed consent applies in that a professional has an affirmative duty to tell a client about the relationship the therapist has with another professional to whom the client will be referred. This is especially true if the referral is going to a spouse or partner. In addition, the referring professional should engage in a process to assist in the decision of whether to refer to a partner or not. This process should be as follows:

1. Ask why is it important that the referral be made to the partner. The answer should be committed in writing. The answer must involve a well-recognized professional purpose.
2. Next, the mental health professional should ask what alternatives are available. The therapist should list the available alternatives. There should not be readily available alternatives if the therapist chooses to proceed with a referral to a partner.
3. The therapist should identify the benefits and liabilities of referring to one of the alternatives.

4. The professional should list the benefits and liabilities of referring to a partner.
5. A session should occur with an objective consultant to discuss the referral issue. If the consultant discourages the referral to a partner, then no referral should occur. The consultant should focus on ascertaining whether any conflict exists in making a referral to a partner and on what problems—ethical, legal, and clinical—might arise if the referral occurs.
6. If the consultant believes the referral is in the interest of the patient, then the professional should request a brief, 15-minute analysis from an attorney who knows the law and ethics of mental health practice.
7. The professional must honestly and genuinely conclude that the referral is in the best interest of the patient.
8. The referral must actually be for a designated need of the patient relevant to psychological or behavioral problems, such as psychotropic medication, psychometric testing, specialized treatment for an identified condition (e.g., cognitive-behavioral therapy for an Obsessive Compulsive Disorder), inpatient treatment, neurological or other physical examination, and so on.
9. The patient must be fully apprised of the relationship between the referring therapist and the professional who receives the referral. Further, the patient must be fully aware of any and all alternatives available.
10. There must be no express prohibition in a professional's relevant ethics code determined either by a case analysis from an ethics committee or in the precise language of the code.
11. There must be no conflict of interest law in the state or federal system where the therapist is practicing which prohibits such a referral. Many laws exist which do apply to employees of state and federal agencies making referrals to a partner who is in private practice.
12. Ultimately the patient must make the choice.
13. Care should be exercised to prevent any conflict of interest from developing during the referral time period which either creates or is likely to create a problem for the patient.
14. All ethical and legal rules must be adhered to during the process.

The process noted above involves self-analysis, objective consultation, strict adherence to law and ethics, and a systematic review of the intended action. Finding an objective consultant is critically important. Many professionals seek consultation from a person whom they know will provide the answer they desire or fail to confront them with any major ethical or legal problems that may arise as the result of the intended conduct. An objective consultant will usually be someone who is paid for services, who has no close relationship with the professional, and where the consultive relationship creates a duty to be honest and objective. Further, the consultant should be experienced and have current knowledge of ethics, law, and community practices where the therapist works (see Appendices B and C on pp. 169-174).

Theoretical orientations of therapists may cause the therapist not to make a referral to a partner, while others are more accepting of such a practice. A strict psychoanalyst would be precluded from making a referral because of the strict boundaries considered necessary for proper treatment. A humanistic or cognitive-behavioral therapist would not have the same theoretical prohibitions to the referral. Although theoretical orientation is never relevant in such ethical matters as sex with clients, sex with former clients, employment of a client, or exploitation in some other way, it is relevant in this arena.

Potential Conflicts

Medication

As noted earlier, one of the most likely scenarios creating a need for a partner-to-partner referral is in the case where a therapy patient needs psychotropic medication. Psychiatrists continue to be in short supply, generally across the United States. Most psychotropic medication used for the treatment of depression and anxiety is prescribed by primary care physicians.

Many primary care physicians are reluctant to prescribe high-powered antipsychotics, including seroquel, geodon, risperdol, haldol, thorazine, stelazine, and especially clozaril. Many general practitioners are also unwilling to prescribe lithium for the management of Bipolar Disorder, particularly when the patient has manic phases requiring control with an antipsychotic such as haldol. Pediatricians are generally unwilling to manage psychiatric disorders requiring medication management of a child, whether the child needs multiple drugs or one medicine. Consequently, patients who need management with medication in addition to psychotherapy find there are limited resources available. The problem is further complicated in the era of managed care where only selected physicians are on a panel to receive referrals from a mental health practitioner. Given the nature of the problem in that there is a lack of resources available to provide medication management for a patient, it seems unreasonable to enforce strict prohibitions pertaining to referrals which may very well cause great harm for a therapy client. No ethics rule in psychiatry, psychology, social work, marriage and family therapy, counseling, or pastoral counseling expressly prohibits referring a patient for medication to a spouse, partner, or close friend, provided all other rules are adhered to in the process (e.g., informed consent). Further, there must not be any exploitation, harm, or confusion in the client, and the referral must not lead to a lack of objectivity in the relationship or be against the law.

Two ways to distinguish this type of dual relationship, besides the fact that there is no expressed prohibition involved, is in the area of harm and professional purpose. Referring the patient for medication to a spouse with informed consent would not result in any appreciable harm to the patient. The patient would be given a choice and, therefore, would enter the referral relationship with his or her eyes open. The couple could not talk to each other about the case unless a release of information was signed by the client. Rather than being harmed, the patient would receive needed medication in a situation where there are limited resources. The important factor to consider is whether there is a primary professional purpose for the activity. Unlike multiple relationships involving sexual contact, employment of a patient, socializing with a client, or borrowing money from a therapy patient, the referral is for a distinct professional purpose directly relevant to the identifiable interests of the client. An activity that causes no harm, does not violate an expressed provision of law or ethics, and is for a professional purpose, is generally going to be ethical and without conflict. Finally, the lack of alternatives is relevant to whether it may be appropriate to refer a client to a partner for medication. If alternatives are available, then the client should be referred to them and not to the partner.

Testing

Another area where a professional may refer to a partner is where the professional is providing psychotherapy and the partner is a psychologist with expertise in psychometric testing. Psychologists are not as rare as psychiatrists or physicians who are experts in psychotropic medication. The State of California has only a few thousand psychiatrists but has approximately 24,000 psychologists and another 1,500 to 3,000 psychological assistants (Board of Psychology [BOP], 2005; www.psychboard.ca.gov). If there are alternatives available, in that other psychologists are in a nearby geographic area that could administer, score, and interpret testing, in order to avoid the appearance of a conflict of interest, the therapist should not make a referral to his or her partner. The problem is that many psychologists do not regularly use psychological testing. In addition, there are recognized subspecialties in the field of psychological tests, such as neuropsychology, child evaluation, memory, developmental disability, and educational testing. Likewise, within the subspecialties, there exists further subspecialization.

There are psychologists who primarily assess children who are suspected of suffering from Attention Deficit Disorder (ADD) or Attention-Deficit/Hyperactivity Disorder (ADHD). In a circumstance where ADD or ADHD is suspected, it may be prudent for an expert in ADD assessment to conduct the evaluation. Likewise, in neuropsychological assessment, psychologists may focus their professional endeavors on epilepsy, malignancies, multiple sclerosis, memory, and head trauma, as well as other areas. A partner who is a psychologist should not be avoided when he or she has special expertise in an area of value to the patient. Just as in the situation with medication management, there should be:

1. A professional purpose in the referral.
2. No law or ethics provision which prohibits the referral.
3. No referral fee.
4. No reasonably available alternative.
5. No harm caused by the referral.
6. Full informed consent of the patient.
7. No other reason that precludes the referral.
8. An objective consultant who concludes that the referral is necessary and appropriate.

It is particularly important that there be no direct financial gain for the therapist who makes the referral. Clearly, there will be indirect financial gain from the referral. That is why the therapist must exercise great care in referring a patient to a partner. However, it is not a perfect world with the best possible alternatives available for the resolution of problems. In a less-than-perfect world, reasoned, goal-directed behavior following principles derived from an ethics code is the next best choice. In referring a patient for psychological testing, reasoning with the above guidance is critically important.

Medical Care

A therapy patient often is in need of medical care, which can range from the most benign, such as a physical examination, to more serious conditions, such as a malignant tumor of the brain. In many areas, there will be alternatives to referring a client to a physician partner.

But in some rural areas or in some subcultures, alternative resources may be unavailable. Some medical specialists are not readily found in most areas of the country, except in large cities where medical facilities are prevalent and often associated with teaching hospitals. Specialists in the areas of, for example, pediatric neurology, rheumatology, endocrinology, neurosurgery, pediatric head trauma, and certain types of oncology, are difficult to find. They are not prevalent in most communities, whereas primary care physicians are not in short supply.

Hence, a referral to a partner who is a primary care physician could rarely be justified, while a referral to a partner who is an endocrinologist could be justified. The difference is in the availability of the resource and the primary professional purpose. When comparable alternatives are readily available, then it is difficult to conclude that the referral to a designated provider was for a primary professional purpose. Consider, however, the circumstance where a mental health professional interviews a client for the first time. The client complains of the recent onset of severe headaches in the upper occipital lobe, as well as blurred vision and balance problems. She has fainted a few times during the past week, and people around her report she exhibits a rather dramatic change in her personality. She notes increased difficulty remembering things in her life. The therapist could wait to make a referral for a physical examination with the patient's primary care provider. Knowing this could take weeks, the therapist calls his partner, who is a neurologist, and describes the patient's symptoms, as well as their recent onset. The partner agrees to see the patient in the afternoon. Regardless of the result in the case, whether it be that the patient has a brain tumor or aneurysm, or suffers from tension headaches, the referral is most likely not unethical. Why? In this case there was a primary professional purpose. In addition, although alternative resources were available, the urgency of the situation from an objective standpoint called for immediate action in the interest of the patient. This illustrates that the general rules should be applied on a case-by-case basis. Some rules, of course, may not be broken, such as the prohibition against referral fees when sending a patient to a partner, or ensuring that the referral is for a primary professional purpose.

Legal Assistance

There are many more attorneys practicing in America today than psychologists or physicians combined. In fact, in California there are more than 150,000 lawyers. In some states, such as Idaho, Montana, or North Dakota, there are fewer attorneys in practice but generally enough to meet the needs of their communities. It would be tempting for an attorney to obtain referrals from a partner who is a mental health professional. The attorney could assist a client in obtaining social security benefits if psychologically disabled, or veteran's benefits, including disability compensation. The attorney could perform estate and trust work, defend clients in criminal matters, and enter into litigation against malfeasant mental health professionals who engage in unethical behavior, whether it be sexual exploitation or harm in another way, including treating vulnerable patients in hot tubs as a means to satisfy the prurient interests of the mental health professional. The attorney could virtually have an entire practice with regular referrals from a partner who is a social worker, psychologist, psychiatrist, counselor, marriage and family therapist, or pastoral counselor. A pastoral counselor could refer numerous church members to the lawyer, as well as actually counseling clients. In exchange, the attorney could refer law clients for therapy or other psychological treatment. As the reader is probably thinking at this point, there are many problems in such a process, and there are subtle differences in referring to an attorney partner compared to the other types of professionals listed previously.

A referral to a lawyer is a problem because, in most communities around the country, lawyers are plentiful. It would not be difficult for a client to find very good legal alternatives in virtually every community. There are, of course, exceptions in extremely rural areas, such as in the northern slopes of Alaska, and in certain subcultures where a prospective client may want an attorney as well as a counselor who is a part of the same general community. This might occur in the gay and lesbian communities. Notwithstanding the exceptions, the fact that readily available alternatives exist means that there is not a necessary argument that could be used by the professional to refer clients to a partner who is an attorney. To the contrary, the availability of other lawyers who could meet the needs of the clients gives rise to a duty not to refer to a partner. Further, the professional could not successfully argue that there was a primary professional purpose in the referral to the partner. Although the client may need legal services, there are others who could provide those services just as well. That leads to the deductive conclusion that the referral was made for a purpose other than to promote the best interest of the client. Given the close relationship between clients and therapists, and the differential power extant in such relationships, there is an increased probability of exploitation on the part of the professional making the referral, as well as for the professional receiving it. A further conflict may emerge if the attorney needs the mental health professional to testify in court on behalf of the client or if it becomes necessary for the mental health professional to be deposed in the client's legal case, write a declaration for the client to obtain benefits of some type, or complete various psycholegal forms to be reviewed by the attorney. The role of the attorney may clash with the therapist in that all attorneys have an affirmative duty to advocate as fully as possible for the legal interests of their clients. In some cases, the legal interest of the client may be in conflict with the therapeutic interest, placing the partners at odds with each other.

There may be circumstances that warrant a limited number of referrals to a partner. However, each of these should be carefully reviewed with a professional consultant who is objective. Otherwise, do not refer a client to an attorney who also happens to be a partner.

Other Types of Professionals

There are other professions where a referral from a therapist may be necessary. These could be physical therapists, accountants, chiropractors, nurses, financial managers, or other mental health professionals with particular specializations such as hypnosis, grief counseling, drug and alcohol treatment, biofeedback, health psychology, forensic practice, or group therapy with a focus on a special area of treatment, such as eating disorders or chronic illness. In dealing with other groups, the rules described above, as well as the thinking process set forth, should be employed by the mental health professional making the referral to a partner. For professions where there are generally ample resources available in most communities, such as chiropractors, physical therapists, accountants, and nurses, a referral to a partner should be considered only if no other comparable resources are available.

Great care must be taken in referring a client to a partner who has a particular mental health specialty. Specialists in the areas noted previously are not commonly found in most communities. There is a clear appearance of a conflict of interest in every referral to a partner. Referring the client to another therapist creates complications in treatment styles, confidentiality, informed consent, patient advocacy, the duty to avoid client harm, competency, and the general duty to have collegial relations with other professionals, on the one hand, and advise them or even report them for unethical conduct, on the other hand.

Inadvertent Multiple Relationships

What about inadvertent multiple relationships involving a couple who are both professionals? These occur rather often, more often than most therapists would like to admit. Suppose a minister in church is married to a physician. The minister provides pastoral counseling as a part of his duties for the church. Unbeknownst to him, several of his clients are receiving medical care from his wife, who is a family practice physician. She has been especially interested in medication for psychological problems and has received extensive training in the prescribing of psychotropic medication. She never medicates patients who are suffering from psychotic disorders, but she often prescribes antidepressants. (In fact, 75% of all antidepressants are prescribed by either family practice or internal medicine physicians.) There would be no way to discover the inadvertent multiple relationships unless an unforeseen circumstance arose or if the client mentioned whom he or she was seeing either for medical care or for counseling. One way the professionals could discover the potential conflict under the above hypothetical scenario is when the client discloses to one provider the identity of the other. It is not unusual for clients to casually mention other health care providers in their lives. Inadvertent multiple relationships must be handled on a case-by-case basis. There is no absolute rule to bring to bear in these cases, other than that the therapist must advocate for and act in accordance with the interests of the client while ensuring that harm is avoided in the process.

Reasons to Refer to a Partner

1. The client needs a particular service provided by the partner.
2. There are no reasonable alternatives available for the client.
3. The referral is for a definite professional purpose.
4. The client, after being fully informed, consents to the referral.
5. There is no harm likely to occur if the patient follows through with the referral.

Reasons Not to Refer to a Partner

1. There will always be an appearance of a conflict of interest.
2. The referral may ultimately cause harm to the client.
3. The referral may be exploitative.
4. There is an increased probability of the client's confidences being breached.
5. The real purpose in the referral may be to meet an economic need of the couple.
6. There are alternatives available that are actually better for the client.

General Rules

Rule #1: Do not refer a patient to a partner.

Rule #2: If you must refer a patient to a partner, first discuss the matter and obtain the approval of an objective consultant.

Rule #3: All referrals to partners must be for a professional purpose.

Rule #4: The mental health professional should not accept a referral fee from the partner for the referral.

Rule #5: The patient should be fully informed about the relationship between the therapist and the partner who will receive the referral.

Most Importantly

Rule #6: Do not discuss the client with the partner unless there is a signed release of information form executed by the client.

Chapter 11

TREATING MULTIPLE MEMBERS
OF A FAMILY AND
OTHER RELATED ISSUES

One area of practice for therapists and for others providing a variety of mental health services is the problem of treating members of the same family. The most common circumstance will occur when a patient is seen for individual psychotherapy by a mental health professional and another member of the family requests individual work. Strict psychoanalytic therapists are precluded from providing individual therapy to members of the same family (Gabbard & Lester, 1995). However, there are certain systems of therapy, notably family systems theorists, who recommend that multiple members of a family be seen in therapy. In fact, treatment of the entire family with a variety of methods, including individual and conjoint work, appears to be one of the hallmarks of family systems therapy (Ackerman, 1970; Erickson & Hogan, 1972; I. Goldenberg & H. Goldenberg, 1980; Luthman & Kirschenbaum, 1974; Minuchin, 1974; and Satir, 1967). The therapeutic emphasis in family therapy is primarily in dealing with those individuals who affect the entire family system (Satir, 1967). A wide range of specific techniques have been developed that are designed to provide treatment which focuses on encouraging family members to change so that the entire system changes (Minuchin, 1974). Of note is that concepts from physics have even been applied to the study of the family as a system in order for it to be better understood (Ebert, 1978a). In addition, an emphasis has been placed upon allowing individuals to become healthier as they function in a healthier family system (Ebert, 1978b).

The ethical problems that arise during this kind of treatment are numerous. One of the primary ethical dilemmas is that in providing marital or family therapy, there may be multiple allegiances demanded or required from the therapist to individual members of the family system. For example, in a family with two parents and three children, each of the five members of the family system may be expecting certain duties and/or allegiances from the therapist to that individual. Many of these expectations of allegiance will be in conflict with other family members' expectations. This creates divided loyalties. Among the first ethicists to deal with this area were Koocher and Keith-Spiegel (1998). They note, "It is most unlikely that the best interest of one client in the treatment group will fully overlap with those of another" (p. 132).

They also discussed the significant problems of conflict that are created with a therapist who sees multiple members of a family. Those areas of conflict were also addressed by Margolan (1982). The conflicts are numerous. One of the primary problem areas is that of confidentiality. When multiple members of a family are treated individually, a therapist is obligated under ethics and law to maintain the privacy of the communications between the two of them. Suppose that the therapist is treating five members of the family in individual therapy as well as in group family sessions. Conflicts may arise when one member of a family, such as a parent, demands to know what has occurred in the therapy of another, most often a child. Given the joint custody laws across the United States, parents generally have a right to confidential medical information about their children. Although there are some exceptions to this rule, a parent can demand, at a minimum, receipt of general information about what has occurred during a therapy session with a child and a therapist. On the other hand, the therapist who is treating all members of the family has an obligation to pursue the best interest of each of those members, both individually and as a group. Consider the following example:

> Ima Snoop is a 42-year-old female who has taken the initiative to bring her family into treatment. The family consists of Ima, her husband, and four children. She is particularly concerned about her 15-year-old daughter, Ineva, who is suspected of smoking marijuana and drinking alcohol. The therapist meets with the entire family as a group once per week. In addition, she provides therapy to the mother and the daughter individually. In the mother's individual sessions, Ima discloses to the therapist that she is particularly concerned about her daughter because she, herself, was an alcoholic in her 20s and was heavily involved in the use and abuse of a wide variety of drugs, including marijuana and methamphetamine. She is terribly afraid that her daughter will follow the same pattern over the next few years. She adamantly prohibits the therapist from disclosing any information about her prior illicit drug use or her alcohol problem. During the family therapy sessions, Ima takes a very strong parental position of no tolerance for the use of any illicit substances. This, of course, is

supported by the therapist. The children in the family sessions report that Ima is a harsh disciplinarian, but they do not disclose sufficient details to require the therapist, under her license, to take any affirmative steps with the state. The adolescent in treatment agrees to talk about her substance abuse problem with the promise from the therapist that none of this will be disclosed to the mother. During the course of therapy it becomes apparent to the therapist that the best interest of her teenage client is to work on the substance abuse problem and to become more independent from her mother. However, based upon the individual therapy with the mother, the therapist concludes that it is in the mother's best interest to have a close relationship with her adolescent daughter. In addition to these problems, the mother demands to have detailed information about the therapy with her daughter. She also demands to review the treatment notes of the therapist on all members of the family.

This is the kind of situation that is often faced by family systems therapists. It may be virtually impossible to resolve the competing interests of the clients. Because all major ethical codes require therapists to engage in activities that promote the best interest of their clients, there will be, at a minimum, a theoretical breach of such ethics for the therapist to focus on the best interest of one client in this family system. Clearly, it would not be in the interest of the adolescent client for the therapist to fully disclose all of the details of their individual therapy sessions. On the other hand, it may not be in the best interest of the mother not to have such disclosure. If other members of the family are seen for individual therapy, an additional problem arises. Notwithstanding the problems with confidentiality and allegiance to one client in particular, there will be a shroud of secrecy about a wide variety of family secrets, in that individual members of the family will be disclosing secrets to the therapist who cannot, in turn, discuss these in family therapy sessions. Although not technically a dual relationship problem, such a process does create dual allegiances and forces the therapist to be involved in multiple relationships with individual members of the family system. The same types of problems exist in group therapy, particularly when a group leader treats group members, both individually and in group sessions.

The problem is further complicated when it occurs in a rural environment. In a rural environment, there may not be a sufficient choice of therapists available to provide individual therapy to members of a family; thus, oftentimes, one therapist alone will provide the family group work. The ultimate ethical requirement, as concluded by Koocher and Keith-Spiegel (1998) is, "A therapist in such situations must strive to ensure that improvement in the status of one family member does not occur at the expense of another" (p. 133). The circumstance noted above creates what Haas and Malouf (2005) refer to as loyalty conflicts. They note that loyalty conflicts may arise when there is difficulty defining exactly who the client is in the treatment setting. In addition, the treatment of several members of a family may prevent the therapist from pursuing his or her ethical duty to advocate on behalf of the client (Morrison, 1986). The problem is further complicated if one accepts the view by Thompson (1990) that one of the duties of a therapist is to promote the autonomy of individual members in treatment. This could be in direct contrast to the goals of family therapy which essentially are to promote better communication among family members and to improve the relationships within the group. This, in and of itself, may be a significant ethical dilemma that may not be resolved adequately (Lakin, 1994).

The problem was of such concern that a number of policies were developed in the CHAMPUS program (now called TriCare). CHAMPUS is the government-sponsored health insurance program for dependents of active duty military members. It is one of the largest insurance programs in the world with an extraordinarily generous mental health benefit. A set of principles were developed for review of insurance where multiple members of a family were treated in therapy. I participated in the drafting of these principles. The policy is presented below (Lieberman & Ebert, 1991, 1993).

In general, combined therapy should be reviewed just as any other mental health service is reviewed in the CHAMPUS Reform Initiative (CRI):

1. Is there a medical/psychological necessity for treatment?
2. Is treatment provided at the appropriate level of care?
3. Is the pattern of service/billing in accordance with generally accepted practice, i.e., is the frequency/intensity of contact with family members appropriate or excessive?

If, in the course of routine review, a question arises about whether a particular instance of combined therapy should be covered, the following principles should be observed:

Principle I: There are circumstances in which care rendered by a single provider to multiple members of a family in multiple modalities of treatment (combined therapy) is appropriate.

Principle II: Such treatment need not be automatically referred to Level III (Peer) Review.

Principle III: A Level II reviewer can approve coverage for combined therapy when he or she finds that it is appropriate.

However, based on the dimensions described in <u>Principle IV</u> below, a Level II reviewer may from time to time question the necessity and/ or appropriateness of this sort of service. In such circumstances, the claim and supporting documentation will be forwarded to Level III for peer review.

<u>Principle IV</u>: Peer review requires that the reviewer is familiar with combined therapy and accepts it as appropriate, given indications for its use. Reviews of such care shall be based upon the dimensions described in <u>Principle V</u>.

<u>Principle V</u>: It is recognized that reviewers must rely on their clinical experience and judgment when considering the necessity and appropriateness of combined therapy. Additionally, they shall consider each claim or treatment episode along with the dimensions described here.

These dimensions are meant as guidelines for review to assure consistency of the review process. They supplement the regulations and guidelines found in the CHAMPUS <u>Operations Manual</u> and the CRI <u>Mental Health Reference Manual</u>.

All guidelines, etc., used to determine medical/psychological necessity for other mental health care, also apply in the case of combined therapy. Specifically, it is noted that CHAMPUS requires that each beneficiary individually receiving mental health services must carry a diagnosed mental disorder (as listed in the DSM-III-R) in order to be covered by the CHAMPUS benefit. In the case of family therapy, this is understood to exclude "counseling" and any therapy that is not specifically directed at the amelioration or elimination of symptoms or dysfunction secondary to such a mental disorder in one or more family members present in the treatment session.

<u>Instances of combined therapy shall be reviewed along the following dimensions:</u>

1. a. Does a clinically consistent and appropriate rationale exist for using the same therapist for multiple members of the family seen in multiple modalities?
    b. Does this rationale follow from the goals and objectives of the treatment plan?

    - Is there a probability that the symptoms and behavioral dysfunctions of the individual members and the family system will be ameliorated by combined therapy? Is this probability enhanced by using a single provider?

- Is there a probability that, in this case, combined therapy will add to or exacerbate symptoms or dysfunctions, or impede the effective completion of treatment of any or all family members?

   c. Is the use of multiple modalities planned and under the clear direction of the therapist useful, or does it reflect counterproductive and counter-therapeutic patterns?

2. a. Are the combinations and permutations of modalities used supported by the characteristics of the case?
   b. Are any of the combinations or permutations of modalities contraindicated?

3. Is the use of combined therapy appropriate to the developmental and circumstantial needs of the individual family members and the family system as a whole?
4. Have multiple modalities been used over a long period of time?

5. a. What are the effects, in this case, of combined therapy on the therapeutic alliances in the family? Does this enhance the trust necessary for successful therapy or does it interfere with that trust?
   b. Have issues such as the limits of confidentiality been discussed? Is the family clear about what communications the therapist will and will not share with any or all family members? Is the therapist aware of his or her limits and policies in these regards?

Many of the ethical dilemmas can be resolved when a family systems therapist does not provide individual therapy to the members of the family. Although there will still be divided loyalties, and although it may be difficult to promote the best interest of all of the clients, it is a purer and less ethically problematic circumstance to separate the modalities of treatment. In looking at major ethical codes and rules on multiple relationships, it is clear that all such codes and rules prohibit multiple relationships where a conflict of interest arises. The circumstances noted above are classic cases where conflicts may arise. The ethics code of the American Association for Marriage and Family Therapy (AAMFT, 2001) is the one code that specifically notes the unique situation that arises in providing marriage and family therapy. Throughout the AAMFT Code of Ethics, there is unique recognition of the differences in providing therapy to more than one individual in a family system. However, as noted above, all major mental health professions require a therapist not to be in a conflict of interest with any individual client.

Reasons to Treat Multiple Members of a Family in Group And Individual Therapy

1. Therapist is functioning in a rural area.
2. After independent and objective consultation, it is appropriate to the situation of the family.
3. The family has limited financial resources and the therapist is able to provide services within the means of the family members.
4. There are no significant conflicts that are obvious at the outset of treatment.
5. There do not seem to be any other reasonable alternatives available.

General Rules

Rule #1: If a therapist provides family therapy to all or several members of a family, he or she should not treat anyone in individual therapy.

Rule #2: If, in the course of providing family therapy, it is apparent that one of the members needs individual treatment, the therapist should refer that member to a colleague for individual psychotherapy.

Rule #3: Prior to entering into individual therapy with a family member who is also seen with his or her family, the therapist should seek objective consultation as to how to proceed.

Rule #4: At any point, if it is apparent that a conflict exists, the therapist must refer either the individual or the family to another provider.

Rule #5: The therapist should not automatically consider providing services to the family as a group and to individual members. (The temptation to do so should be considered a sign of narcissistic defensiveness.)

Rule #6: The therapist must always ensure that the goals of treatment for the family system are communicated to all members of the family in open session.

Rule #7: The therapist must be vigilant to ascertain when any conflicts exist between individual members of the family who are receiving group treatment, and take appropriate steps to resolve such conflicts.

Chapter 12

FORENSIC
MULTIPLE RELATIONSHIPS

An entire book could be written about the complexities of relationships in a forensic setting. Some problems are not unique, while others are. One rather interesting problem has to do with engaging in sexual conduct with someone who is receiving court-ordered forensic services. As noted in Table 5 (p. 38), all major mental health ethics codes prohibit sexual conduct with a client.

Despite the complexities in the forensic setting, until recently, few writers have addressed the issues of multiple relationships. By far one of the most comprehensive chapters on the subject was written by Haas and Malouf (2005) and is entitled "Forensic Mental Health: Practitioners in the Courtroom." The chapter is nine pages long and describes different roles the practitioner may play in the performance of forensic work. Weissman and DeBow (2003) have written one of the newest and most comprehensive works on forensic ethics. They describe two well-known models for dealing with ethical dilemmas in a forensic setting. A more detailed model was developed earlier but will be published in 2006 (Ebert, in press). Much of it is focused upon providing testimony in court, a function that is often a small part of forensic practice. Shapiro (1991) notes that there are many complicated ethical issues in a forensic setting, one of which is defining who the client is. Although Monahan (1980) attempted to answer this question many years ago, the issues are more difficult to resolve than simply labeling a person as a client or not a client. In Shapiro's book, the only reference to the problem of conflict of interest and multiple relationships was in citing Monahan.

Likewise, Appelbaum and Gutheil (1991) devoted a few pages to ethical issues, mostly focused upon specific problems encountered by experts who are testifying in court, such as role confusion created by one side hiring an expert or answering questions during cross-examination in a thoughtful and honest manner. Blau (1984) presents one of the most comprehensive descriptions of ethical issues in the forensic setting. Blau took sections from the 1981 version of the ethics code of the American Psychological Association and briefly discussed how they apply in a forensic setting. Blau identified confidentiality issues as a major area of ethical problems and complexity in forensics, as well as competence, producing high-quality work, and financial arrangements. By far the most detailed writing on ethics in a forensic setting came from Hess (1999) in the seminal work *The Handbook of Forensic Psychology*. Hess has been one of the only writers to address the various role conflicts that exist in the forensic setting. Hess and Blau both address ethical conflicts pertaining to confidentiality and privilege, while Hess goes further in his analysis of conflicts created by the forensic role. Blau, Shapiro, and Hess have all addressed the ethics of providing expert testimony. Likewise, Koocher and Keith-Spiegel (1998) described ethical issues in court primarily as clarifying roles, defining who the client is, clarifying obligations, and presenting testimony in court, as well as use of hypnosis and dealing with child custody matters.

Forensic ethics have improved significantly since the early work of these great psychology writers. In 1992, a specific section was added to the APA Code of Ethics (APA, 1992, Standard 7.0 et seq.), although the forensic section was deleted in the 2002 revision. Division 41 of the American Psychological Association (Committee on Ethical Guidelines for Forensic Psychologists, 1991) promulgated specialty guidelines for forensic psychologists. Guidelines for performing professional services in child custody evaluations were adopted by the APA in 1994, while rules for dealing with test data were outlined in 1996 (APA, 1994, 1995). Vesper (1995) wrote about boundary problems for therapists working with abused clients who are involved in various court actions. There is specific language in the Division 41 Guidelines (Committee on Ethical Guidelines for Forensic Psychologists, 1991) pertaining to dual relationships in forensic practice. The Guidelines provide at III(D):

> D. Forensic psychologists recognize potential conflicts of interest in dual relationships with parties to a legal proceeding, and they seek to minimize their effects.
>
> 1. Forensic psychologists avoid providing professional services to parties in a legal proceeding with whom they have personal or professional relationships that are inconsistent with the anticipated relationship.

    2.   When it is necessary to provide both evaluation and treatment services to a party in a legal proceeding (as may be the case in small forensic hospital settings or small communities), the forensic psychologist takes reasonable steps to minimize the potential negative effects of these circumstances on the rights of the party, confidentiality, and the process of treatment and evaluation. (p. x)

    Probably the first set of formal ethical guidelines applicable in a forensic setting was developed by the American Academy of Psychiatry and the Law (AAPL, 1995). Notwithstanding these great advances, there has been little written about the unique role problems, multiple relationships, and conflicts in forensics. The most recent work in this area demonstrates another evolutionary step in the development of ethical standards for forensic practice. Canter et al. (1994) provide a commentary on the 1992 APA ethics codes. In their book, Canter et al. discuss the importance in clarifying one's role in a forensic evaluation. They also identify conflicts that may be created by prior relationships vis-à-vis testimony in court. The AAMFT does not have a specific section dealing with ethical problems in a forensic setting for marriage and family therapists. Similarly, the NASW code of ethics does not have a section on forensics, nor does the word "forensics" appear in the code. The American Counseling Association *Code of Ethics* does not contain a section on forensic practice issues. As might be expected, the code of ethics of the American Association for Pastoral Counselors does not address forensic issues, as practitioners in this group may be the most unlikely group to deal with the court system. Despite no references to dual relationship standards for forensic practice by the AAMFT, NASW, ACA, and AAPC, there are principles which can be extrapolated to deal with ethical issues in the forensic setting. The next step in the evolution is the identification of the multiple relationship problems extant in a forensic setting.

    Consider this hypothetical example:

    Dr. Tosterone is conducting a court-mandated evaluation in a custody dispute. The parties have already divorced. The couple has two children, ages 10 and 6 years. The order for the evaluation comes directly from a local court, making Dr. T. a temporary officer of the court for the purposes of the custody examination. The evaluation involves a complete custody evaluation in conformance with the APA Guidelines on conducting child custody evaluations (APA, 1994). Dr. T. performs an interview for 3 hours on the mother and father and evaluates each child for an hour and a half. Testing is administered to all parties. The mother and father are given the MMPI-2, MCMI-II, 16PF, Rorschach, Sentence Completion Test, and the Shipley Institute of Living Scale. The parents are asked to complete a behavior checklist on each child, as well as the Personality Inventory for Children. Dr. T. administers a Rorschach, Family Drawing, House-Tree-Person Test, and a Wechsler Intelligence Scale for Children-III to each child. In addition, he reviews extensive data in the case, including school records, pleadings in the case, personnel records of the mother and the father, police reports, and letters of support for each parent. He engages in collateral contacts with two therapists involved in the case and speaks to the teachers of both children.

During the interview with the mother, Dr. T. finds himself attracted to the mother. He has difficulty concentrating and allows himself to engage in various fantasies involving the mother and himself. He is so distracted by his fantasies that he stops the interview and reschedules the mother to return to his office at 9:00 p.m. the next night. After the session, Dr. T. thinks about obtaining professional consultation but decides not to pursue it. Instead he meets the client at 9:00 p.m. the next night. During the second interview the client expresses she is very upset about the divorce. At one point she is so distressed she begins sobbing. To comfort her, Dr. T. stands up from his chair, moves over to her, and embraces her. She grabs on very tightly to him. After they hold each other for 10 minutes, Dr. T. suggests she take the MMPI-2. She does so and completes it at 11:00 p.m. that night. Toward the end of the test the mother complains her neck muscles are very sore. Dr. T. comforts her by massaging her. Shortly after the test is completed the two begin kissing and subsequently engage in sexual intercourse. This process of testing followed by sexual intercourse repeats itself for every other test. Dr. T. elects not to disclose his new relationship with the mother because he is in love with her and wants to marry her. He reads the ethics code, as well as Dr. John Monahan's book on who is the client, and concludes he has not had sex with a client because the evaluation was ordered by the court. A few months later the mother complains about Dr. T. His defense is that his conduct is not prohibited because he did not have sex with a client as the court was his client.

Before the reader stops laughing, it should be noted that the defense offered above is surprisingly not uncommon. It is often put forth because the rules prohibiting sexual conduct with a client most often refer to psychotherapy clients. In fact, other than a complete denial of the allegations, it is the most common defense used in sexual misconduct cases involving a forensic setting. For many years the "Who is the Client" controversy was resolved definitively in favor of the court. That is, the court was considered to be the client and, therefore, deserving of all duties and loyalty emanating from such a relationship. The primary emphasis of this analysis was on dealing with confidential information obtained in the course of a forensic evaluation. Because the court was considered to be the client, it was the court and not the person evaluated that had the privilege or control over the information. This analysis still works in the present day for confidential information but is woefully inadequate in dealing with multiple relationships and conflict of interest issues.

All of the ethics codes of mental health professions have applicable provisions that can be used to guide a professional in avoiding conflicts of interest and multiple relationships. Most professions prohibit involvement in exploitative relationships (APA, 2002, § 1.01 - Misuse of Psychologists' Work, & § 3.08 - Exploitative Relationships; AAMFT, 2001, § 1.3 & § 7.5; NASW, 1999, § 1.06(b); American Psychiatric Association, 2001, § 1(1); ACA, 2005, § A.5.c.; AAPC, 1994, Principle III).

Further, Arcaya (1987) discussed role conflicts as a counter-transference issue, especially when therapists provided court testimony for their clients. He also discussed the problem of conducting an evaluation in what he referred to as a "coercive setting." He identified a helper and a prosecutorial bias, as well as an uncommitted bias, that is often present in a forensic examination. However, Cornell (1987) criticized Arcaya for his use of psychoanalytic terminology and concepts in describing the role conflicts that exist in a forensic setting.

Prior Relationship
With the Judge

No one has written about conflicts that may exist as the result of having a prior relationship with a judge. Some difficulties can arise when this is the case. In fact, in small communities it is not unusual for a judge to become very familiar with forensic practitioners. In many instances the judge may be a friend of the mental health professional. This relationship could cause an actual conflict of interest, if not an appearance of conflict. Judges have general rules of recusal when a conflict of interest exists (Ebert, 1997; 28 U.S.C.A. 455(a), 1997; California Rules of Court, 1997). Only recently have ethicists proposed rules of recusal for mental health workers (Ebert, 1997). Judges are trained to be objective and to put their personal bias and prejudices aside during a case. Of course, they are not always successful. A mental health professional has more difficulty doing the same because there is no training except under the close supervision of a forensic professional. Forensic psychologists often try hard to develop relationships with judges, in part as a function of good marketing.

To date, no professional article has addressed the problems that can develop when the relationship is too close or where it actually or potentially interferes with the outcome of a case, based upon the relationship between the judge and the professional.

The most problematic circumstance occurs when the mental health professional is testifying for a particular side in a legal controversy opposite another mental health professional. This could occur in a criminal, civil, or administrative matter. If the matter involves a judicial decision, such as the admission of evidence, there could be an appearance of a conflict of interest. On the other hand, there is no rule that requires a professional not to have friendships with certain people.

Consider the following scenario:

> Dr. X. Aminer is in charge of court mediation services for the County of Matrimony. He forms a very close relationship with the presiding judge who also assigns all mediators to cases and manages the family law docket. P. Que is a marriage and family therapist who has been a court mediator for several years. She performs services with a couple and discovers that Dr. Aminer engaged in unethical multiple relationships with the couple in his prior work with them. Further, she concludes that his recommendations were based upon bias and were tainted by his personal involvement in the case. When she makes this known to Dr. Aminer, he denies there is a problem and speaks to the judge to have P. Que removed as a mediator. He is successful based upon his relationship with the judge.

This is but one example of what can happen when a relationship with a judge becomes too close. Although many judges are highly ethical and dedicated to functioning as an independent jurist in a free society, some allow their egos to cloud their judgment. It is the obligation of the professional to monitor his or her own behavior and take appropriate steps. The APA (2002) sets forth critically important Principles of Beneficence and Nonmaleficence, Fidelity and Responsibility, Integrity, Justice, and Respect for People's Rights and Dignity that can be used to guide professionals to take the right action in cases. This might involve refusing to take a lucrative case, resigning from a position, or recommending a colleague for a case.

The most common problem with a close relationship with a judge involves dealing with competitors. A close relationship may preclude other more competent professionals from working in a county court setting. A professional making negative comments about others for the purpose of preventing them from obtaining assignment is clearly using the relationship with the judge to violate ethical duties of integrity and collegial relations outlined or implied in all major mental health ethics codes. There is probably a duty to declare the relationship in some instances so all parties may proceed or take appropriate action, such as asking for a new judge or a different evaluator in a case. Candor to the court is an important rule of professional responsibility for lawyers (American Bar Association [ABA], 2003, Rule 3.3, "Candor Toward the Tribunal").

Serving Two Masters

This is a significant problem that has been all but dismissed in forensic settings. Some have thought that the end of the discussion occurred 17 years ago when the client was defined (Monahan, 1980). Monahan's conclusions, although very helpful, do not resolve all of the ethical problems for professionals dealing with people in the court system. In forensic work, there are always at least two parties to whom you may owe allegiance. It may be the court, an attorney, a legal system such as worker's compensation, the law of the state, or the client. This is the conflict discussed, in part, by Arcaya (1987). Conflicts may arise when asked to predict future dangerousness when the result of the prediction may be the death penalty, such as in *Estelle v. Smith* (1981), in which a psychiatrist predicted that the defendant would be a danger to society if left alive. The ethical problems and conflict pertaining to this have been addressed previously (Grisso & Appelbaum, 1992).

Often a professional receives a referral from a court to conduct an evaluation of an individual. Most often this occurs in a criminal setting, but it also occurs frequently in child custody matters where the professional works as a special officer under the umbrella of the court. In some cases, the professional may work for a probation department or a prison, but the professional may also be providing services to an individual who is housed in jail. There are pressures that are imposed upon mental health professionals, both subtle and obvious, and weak and powerful. Using the Monahan approach, the problem can be resolved easily. But the issue is complex. You are providing a service to a human being. Is there not some moral duty to that person to conduct oneself in an ethical manner? Or can a social worker or a psychologist simply ignore the humanity in the person being evaluated and justify engaging in behavior with him or her that would be considered unethical if the person were labeled a client? This is exactly the kind of reasoning and rationale applied by clearly unethical people to defend themselves against sexual acting out in such a circumstance.

It is necessary for the forensic practitioner to understand, at the incipience of employment with a forensic client, that there may be two or more diverse entities demanding conduct that may be in conflict. The psychologist evaluating a defendant to ascertain competency to stand trial is not free to commit a battery on him or her, or engage in sexual contact, even if it is consensual. Nor is he or she free to violate his or her confidences to the general public or perform services appointed by a judge that would be performed incompetently because of a lack of training, education, and experience in this area. The ethical duties of one's profession, in most instances, supersede all other mandates, creating an allegiance to one's professional responsibilities. This allegiance should be so powerful and ingrained into the personality of the professional that the ethics code and its principles take on the role of a person.

Some obvious examples are necessary. A psychologist cannot interview a patient in a jail for the purpose of obtaining the inmate's inner fears and anxieties in order for them to be used by prison guards to torture him or her. The social worker cannot or should not interview a 4-year-old child who is suspected of being abused, using leading and suggestive questions, not to seek the truth, but to have the child admit he or she was sexually abused by his or her father simply because that would confirm the hypothesis of the professional. The marriage and family counselor, who either suffered severe sexual abuse herself or himself or is asked by a police officer only to obtain inculpatory evidence, cannot ethically interview 3- and 4-year-olds in a day care center, using coercive or interrogation tactics, not video- or audiotaped, to incriminate the day care teacher of abuse. The ethical point that must never be forgotten is that although ethical duties may be different when performing an evaluation on a defendant or a witness at the request of your primary client, all professional actions are cloaked in ethical garb which wraps around every act of the professional.

In other words, in virtually all forensic activities there are structural multiple relationships extant by virtue of the system in which you are working. One must be ever vigilant to sort through these issues and analyze them rather than dismiss them by concluding that the human being you are interviewing is not the client. One agonizing example of this in a forensic setting deals with competency to be executed. In *Ford v. Wainwright* (1986), the United States Supreme Court was faced with a unique situation. Alyin Ford was found guilty of murder in 1974 and received the death penalty. He was apparently competent at trial. In 1982, Ford's mental condition began to deteriorate. He became paranoid and thought there was a conspiracy against him involving the Ku Klux Klan and prison guards. He was delusional, believing women in his family were being tortured and being sexually assaulted in the prison where he was incarcerated. Ford was convinced that 135 of his friends were being held hostage in prison. Ford further believed he was the Pope, calling himself Pope John Paul III. A prison psychiatrist diagnosed

Ford as suffering from a severe mental disease tantamount to paranoid schizophrenia. Ford's mental disorder was so severe that he did not know why he was being put to death. Based upon appeals in the case regarding Ford's mental state, the court, in a landmark decision, concluded that a person could not be executed if he did not understand the reasons for the death penalty and its implications. A person must be competent to be executed.

The multiple relationship issue arises in conducting an evaluation as well as in providing treatment. Successful treatment of an incompetent patient on death row would result in the imposition of the death penalty for the patient. Likewise, conducting an evaluation to determine the competency of a death row inmate, depending upon the conclusion, may result in his or her death. This is a professional activity in which there may be six masters: the constitution, one's profession, society, the prison, the state, and the inmate.

Socializing With Forensic Clients

Clearly, socializing with a forensic client would constitute a multiple relationship. However, there are essentially no rules or written standards regarding this. First, it is clear there are different types of forensic relationships. In some, any type of post-case contact would be unethical for the forensic professional and prohibited by the courts. In some circumstances it could constitute ex parte contact which would lead to clear conflict in the resolution of the proceedings. In a custody evaluation, the evaluator is appointed by the court and works as an officer of the court. Any socializing with a client in a custody case would be unethical and illegal. Likewise, in cases where the professional is appointed by the court to perform work pertaining to sanity, competency, sexual or other dangerousness, addiction, probate matters, sentencing issues, and juvenile matters, socializing with a client would clearly be an unethical multiple relationship.

There may be circumstances where it is not unethical. Jury consultants become part of the legal team and are under no prohibition from contact with the client. Any social contact is not likely to have an adverse effect on the client or the professional work performed by the jury consultant. A new area of practice is full trial consultation. The psychologist or psychiatrist may advise the attorneys and the client about various trial strategies drawing from scientific literature. At the end of the case, when all is done it is not unusual for the "team" to socialize with the client by going to dinner. Is this a conflict of interest? Does this cause harm? Does it exploit the client? The answer is probably no. Hence, the precise role of the forensic professional determines whether it is ethical to socialize with the client. Further, what if the client is actually the lawyer or lawyers involved in the case?

In forensic work with the military, lawyers, psychologists, psychiatrists, and other experts such as computer engineers, neurologists, and blood splatter experts travel far from home and often stay near each other. It is customary to work together and socialize, although during a trial the extent of socializing is having dinner together.

Pressure to Produce
A Particular Result

Although it is somewhat of a stretch to consider this category as a multiple relationship problem, it is clearly one of the biggest ethical conflicts facing forensic practitioners. In a forensic evaluation there is always pressure. The adversary system of law in the United States creates an atmosphere of pressure on the mental health professional. Less pressure exists if the court appoints the professional to conduct an independent evaluation in competency, sanity, child custody, competency in a probate matter, determining dangerousness in a child sexual offender, or other related matters. Although there is more reliance on independent appointees of the court, there is still a great deal of work performed by professionals retained by one side or the other. It is not unusual for a defense attorney in a criminal law case to hire a consultant and for the deputy district attorney to do the same. There is either obvious or subtle pressure upon the professional to produce an opinion that supports the side retaining him or her. It is well known that some mental health professionals literally sell their opinions. They always generate a seemingly scholarly opinion in support of the side retaining them.

Often the psychologist or psychiatrist faces the pressure alone and must resist the temptation to acquiesce to the demands of the retaining attorney. This creates a unique type of dual relationship: a relationship where the role itself of a professional demands certain conduct, while the forensic role defined by the retaining attorney demands otherwise. It is a pure conflict of roles with the role definition of a mental health professional on one side and the role definition of an advocate on the other side; following one set of rules likely violates the opposing role requirements. Consider the following example.

Dr. E. Valuator is a forensic psychiatrist working in a city where there are several other forensic practitioners. He is retained by a defense attorney, Ima Winner, in a criminal law case to determine whether the client was insane; that is, whether the client knew the nature and quality of his acts or their wrongfulness at the time of the alleged offenses. The defense attorney is retained by her client, who is very wealthy. Defense counsel is a prominent attorney who rarely loses a case. She pressures Dr. Valuator to conclude the client was insane. Because it is a retained case, Dr. Valuator has been paid a retainer fee of $10,000. Shortly into the evaluation, Ms. Winner calls Dr. Valuator and advises him that she has a few other cases she would like to refer to Dr. Valuator, provided this one works out well. Dr. Valuator concludes that the client was insane and testifies in court about his conclusions. Dr. Valuator's data does not support his conclusion.

It is clear from the preceding scenario that the psychiatrist wrongly interpreted his role with the defense attorney as one requiring a professional opinion desired by the side who retained him. There are slang terms for those who produce the opinion they are paid to state. Unfortunately, the practice is more frequent than one would guess. There is great economic pressure placed on a professional working in a forensic marketplace where there is a great deal of competition. Many attorneys do not want a truly honest and objective opinion, but prefer a professional conclusion in support of the side they represent. To succumb to this is clearly a gross violation of ethics. But as competition and demands to pay debts accumulated in the practice grow, the temptation is ever present to sell out. Selling out is morally and ethically wrong. There is no valid excuse to justify this practice, and those who are guilty of it should be banished from the profession. Yet this is one of the most pressing problems in forensics and one that has received little attention in the professional literature.

The problem has not fully come to light, in part, because more than 75% of all cases, criminal and civil, never come to trial where the flaws in the methodology and opinion are fully exposed in the adversarial system. The mental health professional must stand firm in the face of economic, interpersonal, political, and business pressures to provide an opinion in support of a particular side simply because that side has retained the professional. Some attorneys actually believe that there is an obligation on the part of the professional in the adversarial system to generate an opinion in favor of his or her client. The idea is that the rigorous cross-examination and discovery that occurs will ferret out the truth. Both subtle and obvious manipulation is practiced by an attorney toward the professional. The manipulation may come in the form of berating the opinion of the opposing expert or bolstering the ego of the retained professional with comments such as, "Your work is outstanding," "This is the best evaluation I have ever seen," "You are so much more accurate than Dr. Ebert," or "You are amazing in your ability to identify the exact personality characteristics of the client." It may be genuine praise or abject patronizing. No psychologist, psychiatrist, marriage and family therapist, counselor, social worker, or pastoral counselor has a corner on the market of truth. No one has the keys to all knowledge about another human being. As a matter of fact, there were allegations made in the *Menendez* case that prominent defense attorney Leslie Abrams threatened to fire the evaluating psychiatrist in the case if he did not destroy those portions of his notes that would be damaging to the defense.

Because there is no buffer for the mental health professional in a forensic setting, it is incumbent upon him or her to build structural safeguards. These can come in the form of a consultant with whom the professional meets each week, continuing education, a study group, a consultation group, psychotherapy, a savvy partner in a close relationship, or a senior level professional who serves as a mentor. A person practicing in a forensic setting without a built-in buffer is practicing in dangerous waters. Two of the most extreme instances of this problem were described in published legal cases. In the *Wee Care Day Care* case, a 23-year-old teacher, Margaret Kelly Michaels, was wrongfully convicted of 115 counts of child sexual abuse, physical abuse, and making terrorist threats, and was subsequently sentenced to prison for 47 years (Rosenthal, 1995). The convictions were overturned on appeal and Michaels was set free (*State v. Michaels*, 1993). One individual, calling herself a mental health professional, although unlicensed, conducted interviews of children using her own methodology seemingly designed to convince the children involved that they were, in fact, abused. There was no search for the truth. One child was convinced he was turned into a mouse by Michaels after repeated interviews from a nonlicensed individual who claimed to be a psychologist. This witness constructed a 32-item checklist of symptoms of sexual abuse and seemingly concluded that whatever response a child gave constituted evidence of sexual abuse. This case was written about extensively in an entire issue of the American Psychological Association Journal *Psychology, Public Policy and Law* (Sales, 1995). This was a case where the pressure was to find evidence of sexual abuse, regardless of the truth. The pressure prevailed, and the truth evaporated. Although this was an unusual case given the extreme nature of the facts, all mental health professionals face pressure to generate an opinion compatible with a particular side in a controversy. Ethical individuals withstand the pressure and render professional opinions that are objective, factual, consistent with their data, and reconcilable with current scientific knowledge and theory.

Working for Attorneys
Who Are Friends

It is not unusual to become friends with an attorney while working with him or her during a long and stressful case. Sometimes a professional could spend months or more than a year working on a case with an attorney. If the results of a few cases are successful, it is common for the attorney to request services of the mental health professional in the future. Attorneys are result oriented. It is part of their duty as an advocate for their client. A professional who has favorable results in cases will be in great demand from the attorney involved. The results could come in the form of an acquittal in a criminal case where the professional worked for the defense attorney, a conviction where the professional worked for the prosecuting attorney, a large judgment in a civil case where the professional was employed by the plaintiff's attorney, a determination that no liability or damages existed in a civil case where the professional was retained by the defense attorney, a judicial determination that a worker's psychological problems are severe and are the result of a work-related incident where the professional is hired by an applicant's attorney, or a determination that the worker's problems were attributable to a nonwork condition where the professional was retained by the respondent's attorney.

With good results, people in the legal system emerge who want to be your friend. Still, in other instances, the professional may know the attorney from another setting, such as being a high school classmate, a law school study partner, an acquaintance known through a charitable endeavor, a fellow church member, a co-volunteer, a club member, a neighbor, or through strictly professional contacts in the courts.

One extreme example of how a relationship can obstruct the objective vision of the mental health professional was noted in the case of *James W. v. Superior Court (Goodfriend)* (1993). In 1989 an 8-year-old child, Alicia, was found to be the object of sexual abuse, and her father was accused of the abuse. The child was placed in foster placement and a therapist, Kathleen Goodfriend, was assigned to provide family therapy services. Goodfriend pressured the child to identify her father as the perpetrator. She did this with the knowledge and support of a Department of Social Services (DSS) investigator and a deputy district attorney. Despite knowing that a registered sex offender abducted a 4-year-old girl across the street in May of the same year as the child in question was abused, Goodfriend pressured Alicia to tell her that her father abused her. In fact, Goodfriend, the district attorney, and the DSS worker met in June 1990, and discussed ways to twist the findings of a detective, which tended to implicate the convicted sex offender and not the father. Alicia continually told people around her, including Ms. Goodfriend, that her father was not the perpetrator. She insisted this was the case for over 1 year. Goodfriend repeatedly pressured Alicia to tell her that her father molested her. In fact, Goodfriend told Alicia that if she wanted to go home she must identify her father as the assailant. The collaboration of the three people mentioned previously to implicate an apparently innocent man is virtually unprecedented. Eventually, the truth was discovered and a lawsuit was allowed to go forward against Goodfriend.

Most cases are not as extreme, but working with friends creates additional pressure to produce a finding that supports the case of the friend retaining the professional. There is no absolute prohibition against working with a friend, but there is a prohibition against compromising one's findings because of pressure felt given the relationship one has with the retaining party. The closest rules prohibiting work with a friend appear in the forensic specialty guidelines for psychologists (Committee on Ethical Guidelines for Forensic Psychologists, 1991). Rule IV(D) cautions psychologists in a forensic setting to recognize and minimize conflicting relationships. Rule IV(D)(1) is worded in a rather interesting manner. It provides:

> Forensic psychologists avoid providing professional services to parties in a legal proceeding with whom they have personal or professional relationships that are inconsistent with the anticipated relationship. (p. 659)

AAPL, in its guidelines for forensic psychiatrists, does not directly address the issue, but does require psychiatrists to strive for objectivity in their evaluations (AAPL, 1995, Guideline IV). The 1992 ethics code of the American Psychological Association cautions psychologists from allowing a prior relationship to interfere with psychologists' objectivity, similar to the AAPL rules (APA, 1992, Standard 7.05). In addition, there is a duty not to perform conflicting roles in the forensic setting (Standard 7.03). No set of ethical rules has provided specific guidance involving the practical problems faced by a forensic practitioner who might choose to work with a friend. There should be no absolute prohibition against it, but there may be a need for the buffer zone referred to above to be created by the professional in order to assess, early in the process, when objectivity is compromised.

The other problem that arises in working with a friend, either by blood or by relationship, is the tendency to want to stretch the findings of an evaluation, or push the envelope in terms of court testimony or summarizing the scientific literature on a subject. A good rule to follow is to avoid working with relatives if possible, attempt to avoid working with close friends in a forensic setting, and never work as an expert for a spouse.

Evaluating People
You Know or Who Are Related to You

Evaluating someone you know reasonably well would be a classic conflict of interest and a multiple relationship. The rules precluding multiple relationships that present a conflict of interest apply directly in this circumstance. Performing a forensic evaluation, although probably not as bad as providing therapy to that person, is a conflict of interest. It would raise suspicion by the court that the examination was not objective. It would be totally improper to conduct a custody evaluation where one of the parties is a friend, relative, coworker, or neighbor, and it would be inappropriate to engage in a custody evaluation on a couple known to the professional reasonably well. The model described in Chapter 2 is useful in this case. Friends, neighbors, relatives, and former sexual partners would be part of the prohibited class, thereby precluding a mental health professional from ethically providing services to anyone in the class.

Suppose you have a circumstance where forensic services are desperately needed, the professional knows a party, it is a rural setting, and there are few, if any, other resources available to perform the service. In that scenario, could a provider conduct an exam on a friend or a relative to ascertain sanity, or competency, or fitness to work in his or her present job, or his or her ability to perform the essential functions of the job? The answer is possibly, depending upon the nature of the relationship, the availability of alternatives, the system in which the forensic professional is operating, the other factors noted in the model, and the seriousness of the forensic issue. Most of the relationship types in the prohibited class would be excluded, per se. It would be improper to evaluate one's spouse, or a child, or a current or former sexual partner, a close relative, a student, a supervisee, or a business partner. But under limited circumstances, it may not be inappropriate to examine a distant relative, provided it can be done objectively, or a coworker, provided there is limited daily contact and the system you are operating under condones it, such as is the case in the military. Likewise, evaluating a person with whom there is a distant relationship may be appropriate provided the person is not in the prohibited class. In addition, the evaluator must be ready to acknowledge the prior relationship when questioned about it prior to the evaluation or in court. This process allows a trier of fact to determine what weight the evaluation and subsequent testimony should receive in the case.

Performing Two or More Different Services To the Same Person

Circumstances often arise when an expert is asked to perform more than one specific professional activity with the same client. The most common problem arises when the client is a person seen in psychotherapy and where the court and attorney or the client requests the therapist to perform a forensic service. The problem also arises when a forensic specialist is asked to perform two or more types of evaluations. This conflict may arise in evaluations of competency, sanity, sentencing in civil and criminal cases (fitness, threat), competency to stand trial, and then competency to be executed, to manage one's affairs, or to make medical decisions for oneself. You may provide consultation in a case where you are functioning as an expert witness or assisting the development of cross-examination questions for an opposing expert in a forensic setting where you have evaluated the client in question. There are many other dual roles that arise in a forensic setting. The most common dual role situation is one that is the most problematic. It occurs when a therapist who has been treating a patient involved in a legal case provides forensic services to that person, usually in the form of a forensic evaluation or court testimony. There is no express prohibition against a therapist writing a letter of support to the court for a patient. There is clearly a duty on the part of the therapist to recognize that advocacy is not objective forensic analysis, which is the essence of forensic practice. A therapist has developed a close relationship with a client that may have lasted for years. This relationship undoubtedly causes some of the distance and objectivity necessary in a forensic examination to be diminished. The results of the forensic service may be compromised by the prior relationship with the client. This is a case where there is both an actual conflict and the appearance of a conflict of interest.

There is some controversy about what kinds of different services may be performed by a forensic mental health professional on the same individual. It is not uncommon for a court to request a psychologist to evaluate a defendant's competency and subsequently ask for a separate evaluation of his or her sanity. This problem was addressed recently by Golding and Roesch (1987) as to the ethical duties of avoiding conflicting harm, as well as dual relationships with clients. This position has not changed in more recent work (Roesch et al., 1999). The primary question that must be asked by the professional is whether objectivity will be limited or nonexistent by virtue of a prior relationship with the party now involved in a legal case. Most forensic evaluators believe that a therapist who has developed a close therapeutic relationship with a client is unlikely to possess the requisite objectivity to conduct a forensic evaluation designed to address such critical matters as causation or damages. The dynamics necessary for productive therapy to occur are in opposition to those needed to perform a comprehensive evaluation.

Using the rule described above, a professional should be able to perform an evaluation on a client to ascertain competency, and then subsequently evaluate sanity or provide testimony in a portion of the case, such as in sentencing. A common split in roles in civil litigation involving professional malpractice is to have a professional perform services to assess damages and testify only about the presence or lack of psychological problems in the patient. A separate professional is often retained to deal with the issue of whether the professional violated the standard of care. There is no rule prohibiting a damages expert from also testifying about the standard of care, although the two functions involve distinctly different roles. Sometimes the reason an attorney chooses two professionals is for strategic and not for ethical reasons. It is often better to have more professionals on your side than the opposition. There is no prohibition against the same person performing different functions, such as evaluating competency and sanity, or performing work as a consultant in a case and testifying as an expert. The one area that is problematic is in acting as a therapist and then subsequently performing a forensic evaluation on the same individual. In this circumstance the relationship developed with the patient in therapy may interfere with the objective task of evaluating that person. For therapy to be successful, there must be a level of acceptance of the client and what the client is reporting. The therapist often accepts the client's version of events as being true. The forensic examiner is generally tasked with performing an evaluation to assist in the search for the truth in a legal case. These two roles are virtually incompatible. This issue has been dealt with extensively in the professional literature. Consider the work of Greenberg and Shuman

(1997). The reverse situation arises less frequently. A therapist who has performed objective services as a forensic mental health professional may be asked by the client to provide therapy thereafter. There is no direct prohibition against this, but the professional should be careful. Switching to the role of a therapist may preclude any further forensic involvement in the case. Hence, timing of the switch is everything. The professional should wait until all aspects of the legal case have been resolved, either through trial, settlement, or dismissal. There should be no reasonable chance that the case would in any way require future work of a forensic nature or, if it does, the client should be fully aware of this possibility and of the fact that the professional would not be able to participate in the case as a forensic evaluator. This is part of good informed consent that is critical and ethically mandated in current practice (Ebert, 1997). An example of a conflict that would preclude such involvement would be in a civil case where the evaluator was an independent psychological examiner for the opposing side. It would be inappropriate for the opposing evaluator in the case, such as a defense firm examiner, to provide future psychotherapy services to a plaintiff despite the fact that no future forensic services are anticipated. Doing so might very well create an appearance of a conflict for the lawyers and judges involved in the case. This could have a detrimental effect on the public perception of the profession by third parties. In other words, the behavior of the professional would be causing harm to the reputation of the profession, an important consideration in the desire to practice ethically and wisely.

Advocacy of Your Therapy Client in Court Settings

Another conflict facing many professionals providing therapy to clients involved in a forensic setting is when the client requests that the therapist become involved in court in some way. It is very common for a client who has a worker's compensation or civil litigation case, or even a child custody case, to request that the therapist substantiate psychological injury or damages. Therapists often form a close bond with their clients and want to assist them in court. In doing so, they often make serious errors in judgment by assuming that all information relayed to them by their client is true. One of the biggest mistakes a therapist can make is to write a report or letter to the court that discusses the actions, character, or behavior of a person not seen by the therapist. Consider the following example:

Terry Pust, PhD, is a licensed psychologist providing therapy for a 35-year-old woman who is involved in a divorce proceeding that also entails a custody dispute. She provides ongoing treatment to the woman and has seen the children once. The woman reports multiple episodes of physical abuse by her husband. She also complains that the children were abused by the husband. Dr. Pust writes a letter to the court diagnosing her patient as suffering from posttraumatic stress disorder. She further opines that the PTSD is the result of repeated physical abuse by the husband and that the children are in great danger because of this. The court takes action, on the basis of this letter, to suspend visitation between the children and the husband. Dr. Pust neglects to report that she has never seen nor spoken to the husband.

This is a scenario that occurs all too often. The therapist wants to advocate for her client—an admirable goal. But the advocacy goes too far in that the therapist is making conclusions about facts when she has no possible way of knowing whether they are true or not. It is perfectly ethical and professional to advocate one's well-reasoned opinion once it is derived from an extensive review of the data. In effect, the professional has a mandate to advocate for a scientific and objective assessment of an issue in a forensic context, while the attorneys have a sworn duty to advocate a position, regardless of the objective scientific facts.

A therapist should be suspicious when a client wants him or her to advocate for him or her in court. Not all advocacy is unethical or inappropriate. However, therapists are often in the position to be used as a pawn in legal cases, including those involving child custody, disability benefits for the client, damages from an injury such as an automobile accident, worker's compensation benefits, claims of sexual or racial harassment, licensure status of the client, driving privileges, criminal intent, use of substances while driving, competency to stand trial, veterans' benefits, social security benefits, or issues pertaining to the Americans With Disabilities Act or the Family Medical Leave Act. Given the role of the therapist as one who develops a close relationship with a patient in order to assist in psychological healing or growth, the probability is high to confuse the advocacy required in therapy for that demanded in a legal proceeding. Such acts as making a diagnosis of a patient based solely upon his or her report of a traumatic event can be very dangerous from an ethical and legal standpoint and may seriously harm another person not seen by the therapist. The therapist who diagnoses posttraumatic stress disorder in a patient based solely on an uncorroborated report by either the patient or a parent, in the case of the child, is doing a disservice to all parties involved in the case. This occurs when the qualifying act for the diagnosis is an event without objective evidence and where the only information about such an event comes from a biased party, such as a parent in a child custody dispute. In those circumstances it is better to carefully describe behaviors and words directly observed during personal interviews with certain parties and to always qualify the conclusions. An example of such a qualifying statement is, "I did not evaluate the father in the case, which makes any comments inferred about him to be speculative." A cardinal rule to follow in making statements to the court about one party is to comment exclusively about the party whom you evaluated directly and note limitations in the findings. This approach provides the court with important factual information such that the appropriate weight can be attributed by the court in considering all of the relevant facts and circumstances.

The worst situations arise in child custody cases. These occur when a therapist evaluates one party or a child and a parent and recommends a change in custody based upon the examination. There is no evaluation of the other parent. Family law judges listen very carefully to the recommendations of therapists. They may order a change in custody following a report by a therapist. This could prevent a parent from having access to a child for a substantial period of time despite no direct contact from the therapist with the other parent. There is no proper ethical or legal excuse in a case where the therapist does not carefully qualify his or her recommendations and the lack of objective data to support the conclusions to the court.

Working Against People
With Whom You Are in Conflict

A unique potential conflict of interest or multiple relationship problem arises when two forensic mental health professionals who are enemies are on opposite sides of a case. There is no rule in forensic practice that has addressed this conflict directly, although the rules noted above, which require a practitioner to be objective, provide some guidance. Consider the following example:

Dr. Marry Age is a psychologist who was formerly in practice with Dr. Chee Ter. They practiced together for 15 years, and both became competent forensic psychiatrists. Last year they split their joint practice after a significant amount of conflict. There is a great deal of hostility between them. They work in a geographical area where there are limited forensic resources in mental health. Dr. Age is retained on a case to evaluate a plaintiff who is claiming sexual harassment at the workplace. She was employed in a dentist's office. Dr. Age writes a report concluding that the plaintiff was severely damaged psychologically by her supervisor, a dentist. He made this determination on the basis of using the Beck Depression Inventory and after a 1-hour session with the plaintiff. Opposing counsel called Dr. Ter, in part because she knows there is continuing conflict between Dr. Ter and Dr. Age. Dr. Ter takes the case, and his job is to critique the work of Dr. Age.

This is a case in which no precise rule applies except the general rule in the forensic psychology guidelines requiring objectivity. Clearly, both professionals will need to struggle to remain objective. Is Dr. Ter acting unethically if he takes the case while still feeling resentful toward Dr. Age? Would it matter if Dr. Ter has no more anger or hostility toward Dr. Age? Would it matter if Dr. Ter sought consultation prior to taking the case? Or if he talked the matter over with a therapist or a few colleagues to test whether he could be objective? Would it matter if there were other readily available forensic psychiatrists who would perform the role as a consultant in the case? The answer to all of the preceding questions is yes. Entering into a case where active negative feelings exist, without consultation, without therapy, or without considering referral, raises serious questions about the judgment of the practitioner. However, if there is no active conflict, and an objective consultant can conclude that the psychiatrist or therapist could be objective, there would be no prohibition. The opposing counsel will likely attempt to impeach Dr. Ter during cross-examination on the effect of the prior relationship with Dr. Age. This will be unsuccessful if Dr. Ter's opinion is data-based or one that can be anchored to professional or legal literature as required in forensic practice. Yet impeachment may occur even though the underlying facts used to impeach a witness may be untrue. The lawyer is entitled to cross-examine the witness on the nature of the conflict to show bias by the witness. There is no general rule on this issue, but a forensic professional should be prepared to disclose the adversarial relationship with the opposing expert and take steps in the way of consultation and supervision to prevent the conflict from interfering with the objectivity of the examination in the present.

In a particularly unusual case, I was a forensic consultant on one side of a case in a rural area, while the consultant for the other side was my spouse. Ultimately both of us testified in the case objectively and competently. There was complete disclosure throughout the case, including during the trial. Although not precluded, this type of role conflict is not recommended.

Dual or More Licenses
(Attorney-Psychologists)

An obvious multiple relationship problem may arise when a professional has more than one profession. There are increasing numbers of psychologists who are also attorneys. There are psychologists who are physicians, accountants, ministers, religious officials, nurses, members of Congress, or assistants to powerful legislators and realtors, to name a few. In one instance in California, a person was a house painter and also a therapist. As a part of his advertising for house painting, he offered a few sessions of free therapy for each job he received to paint a home. The temptation exists to move from one role to the other when one has multiple degrees or licenses. Suppose an attorney-psychologist is interviewing a therapy client who happens to be in treatment following the death of a loved one in a hospital. What if the facts turn out to be the best medical malpractice case the professional has ever seen? The temptation would be to stop the therapy and switch to the lawyer mode to earn fees from the great malpractice litigation. To do so would be wrong. It would also be unethical, a conflict, and a violation of the rules involving multiple relationships. A forensic psychologist who is also an attorney, who receives a referral in a personal injury case to evaluate for psychological damages, may be tempted to become the client's lawyer if the damages are high enough. A psychologist who is evaluating a wealthy client who is receiving substandard services from an accountant may want to switch roles and be the client's Certified Public Accountant (CPA). A psychologist who is examining a client following an accident may feel it necessary to become the client's nurse for the duration of the case. Consider the following example:

> Dr. Mo Tivated is a psychologist and an attorney. He has practiced both law and psychology and continues to have a small law practice. He has referred a client for an evaluation in a psychological malpractice case. This happens to be Dr. Tivated's specialty area in law. In talking with the client during the first session, the psychologist discovers the client has been sexually abused by a social worker providing treatment and discovers that financial resources were fraudulently drained. The initial assessment of damages is over a million dollars. A million dollar settlement for the attorney would be $333,000 in attorney's fees. At the end of the session Dr. Tivated asks the client if he could take over representation because the other client's lawyer is reported to be inexperienced in this area of law. The client agrees.

This is a classic example of a multiple relationship that is a conflict of interest. The psychologist would be functioning in two separate roles with the client, because the initial reason for contact with the client was for the expressed purpose of performing psychological services. The first contact generally sets the primary relationship with the client. One cannot perform services for a client requiring two different licenses. This does not mean that an evaluator cannot use knowledge obtained in the course of study about a field to benefit the client. The person cannot perform two distinct roles with the same client. The physician cannot be the evaluator and also treat the accident victim who sustained a broken leg; the CPA cannot complete the taxes for a client he or she is evaluating as a psychologist. The psychologist cannot allow himself or herself to perform engineering work on the home of a client. The roles must remain separate for the integrity of the system to survive. The rule applied in these circumstances is simple: *Only perform services with one license for a client. Never perform services requiring two professional roles with the same client.*

When Your Friend or Consultant Is Involved in the Case

Another variation on the same theme is where there is a prior close relationship with someone associated in the case. The evaluator could be a friend of a therapist providing services in a case or an associate of another consultant in the case. Suppose a client is receiving services from a friend or a spouse and is sent for an independent evaluation pursuant to a worker's compensation claim. In a large urban area where there are many forensic practitioners, it would be prudent to refer the client elsewhere. But would a relationship with a friend or with one's spouse necessarily lead to a biased result? The answer is no, although the forensic professional must be very careful in that the legal system is dependent upon objectivity, fairness, and justice. Any relationship that causes a question regarding one of the three is, at least, creating an appearance of a conflict. Should a conflict arise, such a conflict may be overcome with evidence.

In some cases, colleagues who respect each other or who may be friends at some level may be called upon to take opposing positions in a case. Should the relationship between the two experts prevent them from working on the same case on opposite sides? Probably not. Provided there is full disclosure at the outset, no rule prohibiting conflicts or dual relationships would be broken. The experts must be sure not to discuss the case when they meet outside the forensic forum. Each expert must be certain that the relationship with the opposing expert will not in any way adversely affect the work done in the case or the opinions generated for the courts.

Multiple Roles and Conflicts
In a Prison Setting

The employment setting with the most structural conflicts and designated multiple relationships is that of a correctional center. In prisons, mental health professionals provide a variety of forensic services, including therapy to prisoners, evaluation of inmates, parole determinations, assessment of future dangerousness, determinations of suicide potential, educational programs, competency to stand trial assessments, competency restoration programs, diagnosis of mental disorders for the purpose of use of psychotropic medication, competency to be executed evaluations, death penalty sentencing evaluations, participation in involuntary treatment, and medication determinations, which often result in a hearing for the prisoners (see *Riese v. St. Mary's Hospital & Medical Center*, 1987; also see *Keyhea v. Rushen*, 1986), sanity restoration treatment, assessment of the need for certain levels of restraint needed for the prisoner, as well as deciding whether a person needs restraint and seclusion and for how long. Other forensic services not mentioned above may also be provided by mental health professionals.

Classic conflict exists when the professional provides therapy to an inmate/patient. Therapy involves the development of a close, somewhat intimate relationship with a patient. In order for this to happen, the client must develop a measure of trust in the therapist. In private practice, this occurs much more easily because the client hires the therapist and the involvement of third parties is limited, except in the case of some managed care programs. No private setting creates as much of a conflict in roles as that of a prison or a jail. In jail, the therapist is hired by the government that played a role in placing the client behind bars. But, if not for the government funds, the therapist would not be in the prison. The prisoner, in most instances, never pays for services. In some jails, there are experimental programs to charge a small co-pay to inmates in the amount of approximately $3.00. The trust level must certainly be compromised and therapeutic benefit limited by the fact that the trust between therapist and client is potentially irreparably wounded. Role conflict is virtually built into almost every job in the prison setting. A staff member who participates in a take-down and restraint of an inmate may have difficulty gaining the requisite trust necessary to conduct meaningful therapy thereafter. A staff member who orders seclusion for an inmate may be viewed with suspicion by the inmate during subsequent sessions.

Some institutions have instituted policies that shelter a therapist from potentially conflicting roles by having others conduct restraint, seclusion, punishment, restrictions, or involuntary medication. This is critically important because of the structural conflicts built into the setting.

Rules

Rule #1: Be ever vigilant for role conflicts in a forensic setting.

Rule #2: Perform only one primary role in a forensic case.

Rule #3: Never act under the authority of two licenses for the same person in a forensic case.

Rule #4: Always inform clients and parties of potential conflicts of interest.

Rule #5: Seek consultation when pressured to engage in an unethical act by an attorney.

Rule #6: Always keep in mind the affirmative duty to the ethics of the profession.

Rule #7: Be careful in accepting cases in which a person in the case is in conflict with you.

Rule #8: Resign from a case if ethical standards cannot be practiced or reconciled within the case.

Rule #9: Do not comment upon the mental state of someone you have not evaluated personally.

Rule #10: If you are a therapist, never be in a legal case as a forensic expert for one of your clients.

Chapter 13

CONCLUSION

Our journey is essentially over, yet beginning; that is to say, the book is finished, yet the applications to professional practice for the remainder of your career are beginning at this point. There are numerous essential rules for dealing with multiple relationships in an ethical manner. The foundation for appropriate action in these issues, as with all ethical dilemmas, is virtue. That is, it is incumbent upon you to make a deep and passionate commitment to virtuous practice. Virtue, or moral excellence, is the starting point for all ethical conduct in the mental health professions. Benjamin Franklin spoke and wrote of virtues to guide humankind in living their lives in an orderly, morally appropriate manner (Rogers, 1996). Many of the virtues discussed by Franklin apply to the ethical principles of multiple relationships in current practice; these include Order, Resolution, Industry, Sincerity, Justice, Tranquility, and Humility (Rogers, 1996). Swanton (2003) defines a virtue as:

> A good quality of character, more specifically a disposition to, or acknowledge, items within its field or fields in an excellent or good enough way. (p. 19)

Virtuous action in mental health is the deep commitment toward guiding one's conduct in a manner consistent with the very best in human behavior and applying the tools of the profession with the betterment of humankind as a guiding principle and meeting one's own needs as an afterthought. It entails recognition of fundamental and general principles of moral behavior and thought as well as understanding and applying those principles in mental health practice. The best aspect of virtue occurs when it is integrated into the personality of the professional and becomes a central component of all functioning, not just professional activities. For multiple relationship ethics to be understood and practiced most proficiently, virtue forms the basis for all action, and the professional seeks to perform ethically because it is the right thing to do, not to avoid punishment. It entails reaching Kohlberg's (1981) highest level of moral development.

The next step, which is of critical import, is understanding the specific rules of action when a multiple relationship arises. As you have studied in this book, there are many detailed rules of conduct when it comes to dealing with multiple relationships. Some are very easy to understand and involve little debate. For example, the rule against sexual contact with clients is clear and without ambiguity. Others are more complex, such as attending a large social gathering in a rural community. In this book we examined the many facets of multiple relationships, including sex with clients, sex with prior clients, supervision, teaching, professional relationships, social encounters with clients, inadvertent multiple relationships, and forensic issues.

Although it is important to learn and practice the general rules based upon conservative principles, it is also important to have an analytical model to bring to bear in dealing with multiple relationship problems that arise in practice where the rules are not so clear. The models presented in this text can be used to approach new situations with reason and to exclude emotional variables. It is the use of reasoned analysis conducted in an objective setting with objective consultants, if necessary, that will lead to ethical choices regarding multiple relationship problems. The primary model in this book may appear complex, but it is not. It calls for reasoned thought to determine whether there is likely to be any harm to the client, exploitation, create a lack of objectivity in the professional relationship, limit the future choices of the client and therapist, and ultimately create conflict in the relationship. The Ebert model (see Figure 1, pp. 28-30) identifies certain multiple relationships that are unethical, per se. These are referred to as being in the prohibited class. When one of these circumstances arises, the model calls for not providing services in some instances with the individual in question or discontinuation of the prohibited relationship. But there are many occasions when things are not so easy. When the relationship is outside the prohibited class, then further analysis is required. This book assists you in moving through the steps when the rules do not cover the particular problem situation presented to the professional.

In addition to the above, this book examined in detail several areas that have been left out of professional discussions on multiple relationships. For example, the section on social contact deals with actual situations that arise for many mental health professionals. Circumstances such as attending a funeral or a wedding are rather complex, and depend on such variables as virtue, boundaries, distance in the relationship, and theoretical orientation of the professional.

In many respects this work presented you with a regression equation for success. The variables in the equation entailed virtue plus an understanding of the precise rules applicable to the situation plus maintaining appropriate boundaries given the totality of the circumstances and adherences to relevant laws. In addition, the provider must be ever vigilant to the emergence of a multiple relationship issue. In areas where there are no precise rules or regulations or a specific ethics code provision on the topic, then a method of analysis must be applied to lead to the right course of conduct. In the form of an equation it would look like this:

Virtue + Rules + Boundary Maintenance + Laws + Reason and Analysis = ETHICAL CONDUCT

Some variables will change in the equation. Specific laws, ethical standards, and general rules may change, but virtue and boundary control will not. Virtue plus use of the analytical models in this book will lead to sound ethical decisions and safe practice. Safe practice leads to the promotion of client health, the ultimate goal of mental health practice, as well as sound sleep at night.

For the first time, one of the areas covered in an ethics discussion are multiple relationships in forensic settings. Although most readers of this book are not forensic practitioners, most will likely encounter a situation in which they are forced to deal with the legal system, whether it is in a divorce or custody matter, a work stress situation requiring statements about the nature and extent of a client's limitations on the job, or responding to a subpoena for records. The analytical model and the rules applicable to forensic practice may be used to avoid dealing with the court or to clarify the ethical limitations of one's involvement in a case.

Another new area covered in this book is inadvertent multiple relationships. It is quite easy to find yourself in a multiple relationship without anticipating or predicting it. Unforeseen situations involving a multiple relationship problem may arise. Use of reasoned analysis plus virtue will assist you in either discontinuing secondary relationships or in eliminating the primary professional relationship in the most ethical and stress-free manner for the client.

It has been said that you can teach ethical rules but not judgment. In many respects that is true. An individual who is impaired or suffers from a serious personality disorder will make bad choices regardless of his or her knowledge of the rules, ethical principles, or laws. This book takes a very complex and common ethical problem and assists you in guiding yourself through resolution. You may use the content of this book to assist your colleagues regardless of whether you are in a formal supervision or consultation relationship with them. You may also consider fellow professionals with multiple relationship problems to be good friends. Now, armed with the conservative rules, adding commitment and virtue, maintaining appropriate boundaries, and using the models regularly will help you resolve ethical dilemmas and keep you striving to assist those who seek your professional services toward excellence in every aspect of professional practice.

APPENDICES

Appendix A

PROFESSIONAL ASSOCIATION ADDRESSES*

American Association for Marriage and Family Therapy
112 South Alfred Street
Alexandria, VA 22314-3061
(703) 838-9808
www.aamft.org

American Association of Pastoral Counselors
9504A Lee Highway
Fairfax, VA 22031-2303
(703) 385-6967
www.aapc.org

American Bar Association
321 North Clark Street
Chicago, IL 60610
(312) 988-5000
www.abanet.org

American Counseling Association
5999 Stevenson Avenue
Alexandria, VA 22304
(800) 347-6647
www.counseling.org

---

* All readers of this book are strongly encouraged to join a professional association. Associations provide valuable information to members that can assist in promoting ethical conduct. Please write to the associations above to receive a copy of their respective codes of ethics.

American Psychiatric Association
1000 Wilson Boulevard, Suite 1825
Arlington, VA 22209-3901
(703) 907-7300
www.psych.org

American Psychological Association
750 First Street, NE
Washington, DC 20002-4242
(202) 336-5500
www.apa.org

National Association of Social Workers
750 First Street, NE, Suite 700
Washington, DC 20002-4241
(202) 408-8600
www.naswdc.org

Appendix B

GUIDELINES FOR SELECTING AN ATTORNEY CONSULTANT

Qualifications

1. Make sure the attorney has either a Juris Doctor (JD) degree or a Bachelor of Legal Literature (LLB).
2. Some attorneys may have an LLM* (Master of Legal Literature) degree or a Doctor of Jurisprudence (JSD), which indicates advanced education in a particular area.

   * Ask what was the specialty area for the LLM or JSD degree. Some attorneys specializations are taxation, business, environmental law, international law, criminal law, family law, securities law, personal injury, bankruptcy, administrative law, and so on. To find an attorney who will assist you and be of the most help with mental health issues, look for attorneys who specialize in family law, personal injury, or administrative law with special expertise in mental health issues.

3. A small number of attorneys across the country have an LLM with a specialization in mental health law. This would be an ideal educational background for a consultant to have. Others will have an LLM degree in health law with an area of specialization in mental health law.
4. Ideally the attorney would have a degree in one of the behavioral sciences at the graduate level. This includes the Master of Arts, Master of Social Work, Medical Doctor with a specialization in psychiatry, or PhD in psychology. Such programs include:

- PhD — Clinical Psychology
- MA — Counseling
- MA — Psychology
- MA — Marriage, Family, and Child Counseling
- MSW — Clinical Social Work
- MD — with residency in psychiatry
- MA — Educational Psychology
- PhD — Educational Psychology
- EdD — Educational Psychology
- MFT — Marriage and Family Therapist

5. Ideally the attorney is licensed in one of the mental health professions. These include Psychology, Social Work, Mental Health Counselor, Medicine with a Board Certification in Psychiatry, and Marriage, Family, and Child Therapy.
6. Preferably the attorney obtained legal training at a school accredited by the American Bar Association.

Experience

1. The attorney should have been practicing for a minimum of 5 years.
2. The attorney should have familiarity with administrative law, because all licensing board cases are handled under administrative law rules. Administrative law is very different from that of other types, in that the normal rules of evidence are relaxed, there are no juries, and procedures are governed by special statutes often referred to as Administrative Practice Acts.
3. The attorney should be familiar with the rules of civil procedure of the jurisdiction where the mental health law issue will be heard. This could be the state where the mental health professional is licensed. The attorney should be familiar with the rules of motion practiced in the forum where the issue might be heard.
4. The attorney should have experience consulting with mental health professionals. The experience could come in the form of direct consultation to professional organizations such as state associations, national associations, or local professional groups. Or it could come in the form of consulting directly with professionals, such as university counseling centers, individual professionals, group practices, or professional corporations. Some of the best attorneys with knowledge in mental health law are practicing in law firms that defend malpractice claims against mental health professionals. Others have developed a practice in administrative law and have defended mental health professionals in licensing board actions. Some may have defended professionals

in ethics committee hearings, although as of this date the NASW does not allow attorneys to represent social workers in their national ethics committee hearings.

A social worker who is charged with a violation of the ethics code should seek an attorney skilled in administrative, constitutional, and personal injury litigation as well as advanced civil procedure. There is a very special expertise needed in consulting with mental health professionals. An attorney with a general practice or a specialty practice with no experience in mental health law will be virtually useless.

5. A specialist in mental health law will almost never be listed in a telephone directory. It is best to request referrals from colleagues. Consider asking the following:

   - A friend.
   - Your local professional organization.
   - Your state professional organization.
   - An attorney who is a friend.
   - The licensing board in the state where you are licensed; ask them who they think is a good attorney. (I have often given out the names of the very best lawyers who come before the Board of Psychology to those who are in trouble because I, like many other licensing board members, believe in due process and the right of the professional to receive the best defense possible.)
   - Your national professional organization, although they do not keep lists of mental health law experts in each state.
   - The American Bar Association Commission on Mental and Physical Disability Law.
   - Your professional liability insurance carrier.
   - The author of this book (as a last resort).

6. Fees will be relatively expensive for consultation and legal work. Fees range from $175 to $250 per hour for a mental health law consultant. Remember, though, that fees are negotiable. One of the best ways to negotiate a fee reduction is to contract with the attorney for a year-long retainer agreement. You pay, for example, $2,500 as a retainer fee at the beginning of the year, but you contract for a reduced fee of anywhere from $125 to $150 per hour for services across the entire year. Incidentally, the retainer fee must be placed in a client trust fund and cannot be used until the lawyer has performed services for you. Make sure the agreement is in writing, although the State Bar now requires written fee agreements

between lawyers and clients. Another method of negotiating a fee reduction is to gather a group of trusted colleagues together and approach the attorney for a group rate. Also, in the year-long retainer agreement, negotiate for access at any time during the day or evening. Often problems arise after 5:00 p.m. or on the weekends. It is important to be able to reach your lawyer during those times of crisis. Finally, ask about back-up or paging availability for your lawyer. Your lawyer should have some type of back-up system in place similar to what is required of you in your professional practice.

7. Make sure you are comfortable with your lawyer. Make an appointment to be sure you can work with the person. You will be consulting your lawyer on anxiety-provoking issues. It is essential that you are emotionally comfortable to the extent that you can be totally honest and candid in your reports to him or her of your problem issues.

8. Call the State Bar of the state where the lawyer is practicing to determine whether he or she still has a license to practice. Also, ask about prior disciplinary action against the lawyer. This is public information. Remember to call the licensing board of the state where the lawyer has a license in a mental health specialty. Ask for information about discipline of the individual to ascertain whether there have ever been any sustained charges against him or her.

9. Some lawyers are law professors with extensive knowledge in mental health law issues. This type of person would be an ideal consultant provided he or she has an active license to practice. Some law professors place their bar license on inactive status while they are teaching.

10. Make sure your lawyer consultant does not have a serious mental disorder, substance abuse problem, or severe personality disorder. Some lawyers do have those problems, and you do not want to have such a problem lawyer as your consultant.

11. A former deputy attorney general who worked in the area of licensing law is an excellent choice, because the person has experience in the law and practice issues pertaining to administrative law.

Appendix C

HOW TO SELECT A
NONATTORNEY CONSULTANT

1. The consultant should have several years of clinical experience. Five years experience is a minimum, although a newly graduated mental health professional may have some extraordinary insight into practice issues.
2. The consultant should be well versed in professional ethics.
3. The consultant should not be a friend. A friend is less likely to tell you that you are making a mistake or that you are wrong. The friend may give you the impression that you are doing the right thing in a situation when you are doing just the opposite.
4. Members or past members of an ethics committee may be appropriate consultants.
5. The person should understand the licensing laws governing your practice.
6. Ideally the consultant would be actively involved in teaching various topics in mental health.
7. The consultant should provide consultation as part of his or her practice, not just do it once as a favor for you.
8. A person who has sat on a licensing board may make an ideal consultant.
9. The consultant should live a lifestyle and practice professionally consistent with ideal ethical principles.
10. Licensing boards usually know of the best consultants in the state. It is appropriate to ask them whom they recommend.
11. National and state professional associations both should be able to recommend consultants.

12. Talk to your professional colleagues. Ask them whom they have used as consultants.
13. Authors of books on consultation or ethics are appropriate consultants.
14. Define the issue; if it involves a technical area of practice, make sure your consultant knows the area (e.g., Dissociative Identity Disorder and off-site therapy; use of the MCMI-III in a custody case).

REFERENCES

Ackerman, N. W. (1970). *Family Process*. New York: Basic Books.

Allen, G., Szollos, S., & Williams, B. (1986). Doctoral students' comparative evaluations of the best and worst psychotherapy supervision. *Professional Psychology: Research and Practice, 17,* 91-99.

American Academy of Psychiatry and the Law (AAPL). (1995). *Ethical Guidelines for the Practice of Forensic Psychiatry*. Bloomfield, CT: Author.

American Association for Counseling and Development. (1988). Ethical standards. *Journal of Counseling and Development, 67*(1), 4-8.

American Association for Marriage and Family Therapy (AAMFT). (2001). *Code of Ethics*. Washington, DC: Author.

American Association of Pastoral Counselors (AAPC). (1994). *Code of Ethics*. Washington, DC: Author.

American Bar Association (ABA). (2003). *Model Rules of Professional Responsibility* (Rule 3.3, Candor Toward the Tribunal). Chicago, IL: Author.

American Counseling Association (ACA). (2005). *ACA Code of Ethics*. Washington, DC: Author.

American Psychiatric Association. (2001). *The Principles of Medical Ethics With Annotations Especially Applicable to Psychiatry*. Washington, DC: Author.

American Psychological Association. (1958). Ethical standards of psychologists. *American Psychologist, 18,* 279-282.

American Psychological Association. (1977, March). Ethical standards of psychologists. *APA Monitor*, pp. 22-23.

American Psychological Association. (1979). *Ethical Standards of Psychologists*. Washington, DC: Author.

American Psychological Association. (1992). Ethical principles of psychologists and code of conduct. *American Psychologist, 47,* 1597-1611.

American Psychological Association. (1994). Report of the ethics committee, 1993. *American Psychologist, 49,* 659-666.

American Psychological Association. (1995). Report of the ethics committee, 1994. *American Psychologist, 50,* 706-713.

American Psychological Association. (2002). Ethical principles of psychologists and code of conduct. *American Psychologist, 57,* 1060-1073.

American Psychological Association, Committee on Professional Standards. (1987). *Casebook on Ethical Principles of Psychologists.* Washington, DC: Author.

Appelbaum, P. S., & Gutheil, T. G. (1991). *Clinical Handbook of Psychiatry and the Law* (2nd ed.). Baltimore, MD: Williams & Wilkins.

Arcaya, J. M. (1987). Role conflicts in coercive assessments: Evaluation and recommendations. *Professional Psychology: Research and Practice, 18*(5), 422-428.

Bader, E. (1994). Dual relationships: Legal and ethical trends. *Transactional Analysis Journal, 24*(1), 64-66.

Bates, C. B., & Brodsky, A. M. (1989). *Sex in the Therapy Hour.* New York: Guilford.

Behnke, S. (2004). Multiple relationships and APA's new ethics code: Values and applications. *Monitor on Psychology, 35*(1), 66-68.

Bersoff, D. N. (2003). *Ethical Conflicts in Psychology* (3rd ed.). Washington, DC: American Psychological Association.

Blau, T. H. (1984). *The Psychologist as Expert Witness.* New York: John Wiley.

Blevins-Knabe, B. (2003). The ethics of dual relationships in higher education. In D. N. Bersoff (Ed.), *Ethical Conflicts in Psychology* (3rd ed., pp. 239-241). Washington, DC: American Psychological Association.

Borys, D. S. (1992). Nonsexual dual relationships. In L. VandeCreek, S. Knapp, & T. L. Jackson (Eds.), *Innovations in Clinical Practice: A Source Book* (Vol. 11, pp. 443-454). Sarasota, FL: Professional Resource Press.

Borys, D. S. (1994). Maintaining therapeutic boundaries: The motive is therapeutic effectiveness, not defensive practice. *Ethics and Behavior, 4,* 267-273.

Borys, D. S., & Pope, K. S. (1989). Dual relationships between therapist and client: A national study of psychologists, psychiatrists, and social workers. *Professional Psychology: Research and Practice, 20,* 283-293.

California Business and Professions Code. Section 729. (1995).

California Civil Code. (1994). Section 43.93(b) (2).

California Code of Regulations, Title 16, § 1387 et seq. (2001).

California Government Code. (2001). Section 89503.

California Rules of Court. (1997).

Canter, M. B., Bennett, B. E., Jones, S. E., & Nagy, T. F. (1994). *Ethics for Psychologists: A Commentary on the APA Ethics Codes.* Washington, DC: American Psychological Association.

Cavallara, M. L., & Ramsey, M. L. (1988, April). Ethical issues in gerocounseling. *Counseling and Values, 32,* 221-227.

Clarkson, P. (1994). In recognition of dual relationships. *Transactional Analysis Journal, 24*(1), 32-55.

Cohen, E. D., & Cohen, G. S. (1999). *The Virtuous Therapist.* Boston, MA: Brooks/Cole Wadsworth.

Committee on Ethical Guidelines for Forensic Psychologists. (1991). Specialty guidelines for forensic psychologists. *Law and Human Behavior, 15*(6), 655-666.

Cornell, D. G. (1987). Role conflicts in forensic clinical psychology: Reply to Arcaya. *Professional Psychology: Research and Practice, 18*(5), 429-432.

Ebert, B. W. (1978a). Homeostasis. *Family Therapy, 5*(2), 171-175.

Ebert, B. W. (1978b). The healthy family. *Family Therapy, 5*(3), 227-232.

Ebert, B. W. (1997). *Informed Consent. Board of Psychology Update-III.* Sacramento, CA: Board of Psychology.

Ebert, B. W. (2002). Dual-relationship prohibitions: A concept whose time never should have come. In A. Lazarus & O. Zur, *Dual Relationships and Psychotherapy* (pp. 169-211). New York: Springer.

Ebert, B. W. (in press). Analytical model for dealing with forensic ethical dilemmas.

Edelstein, L. (1943). *The Hippocratic Oath: Text, Translation, and Interpretation.* Baltimore, MD: Johns Hopkins Press.

Erickson, G. D., & Hogan, T. P. (1972). *Family Therapy: An Introduction to Theory and Technique.* Monterey, CA: Brooks/Cole.

Estelle v. Smith, 451 U.S. 454 (1981).

Federal Securities and Exchange Act. (1934). United States Code Annotated.

Ford v. Wainwright, 477 U.S. 399, 106 S.Ct. 2595 (1986).

Gabbard, G. O. (Ed.). (1989). *Sexual Exploitation in Professional Relationships.* Washington, DC: American Psychiatric Press.

Gabbard, G. O. (1994). Reconsidering the American Psychological Association's policy on sex with former patients: Is it justifiable? *Professional Psychology: Research and Practice, 25*(4), 329-336.

Gabbard, G. O., & Lester, E. P. (1995). *Boundaries and Boundary Violations in Psychoanalysis.* New York: Basic Books.

Gabbard, G. O., & Pope, K. S. (1989). Sexual intimacies after termination: Clinical, ethical and legal aspects. In G. O. Gabbard (Ed.), *Sexual Exploitation in Professional Relationships* (pp. 115-127). Washington, DC: American Psychiatric Press.

Gifis, S. H. (1984). *Law Dictionary*. New York: Barrons.

Goldenberg, I., & Goldenberg, H. (1980). *Family Therapy: An Overview*. Monterey, CA: Brooks/Cole.

Golding, S. L., & Roesch, R. (1987). Defining and assessing competency to stand trial. In I. B. Weiner & A. K. Hess (Eds.), *Handbook of Forensic Psychology* (2nd ed., pp. 395-437). New York: John Wiley.

Gottlieb, M. C., Sell, J. M., & Schoenfeld, L. S. (1988). Social/romantic relationships with present and former clients: State licensing board actions. *Professional Psychology: Research and Practice, 19*, 459-462.

Greenberg, S. A., & Shuman, D. W. (1997). Irreconcilable conflict between therapeutic and forensic roles. *Professional Psychology: Research and Practice, 28*(1), 50- 57.

Grisso, T., & Appelbaum, P. S. (1992). Is it unethical to offer predictions of future violence? *Law and Human Behavior, 16*, 621-633.

Gutheil, T. G., & Gabbard, G. O. (1993). The concept of boundaries in clinical practice: Theoretical and risk management dimensions. *American Journal of Psychiatry, 150*, 188-196.

Haas, L. J., & Malouf, J. L. (2005). *Keeping Up the Good Work: A Practitioner's Guide to Mental Health Ethics* (4th ed.). Sarasota, FL: Professional Resource Press.

Hatcher, E. R. (1993, June 4). Firm boundaries: No exceptions. *Psychiatric News*, p. 23.

Herlihy, B., & Corey, G. (1992). *Dual Relationships in Counseling*. Alexandria, VA: American Association for Counseling Development.

Hess, A. K. (1999). Serving as an expert witness. In I. B. Weiner & A. K. Hess (Eds.), *The Handbook of Forensic Psychology* (2nd ed., pp. 521-559). New York: John Wiley.

Hunniecutt v. The State Bar of California, 44 Cal.3d 362, 748 P.2d 1161 (1988).

In re John Spurr. (1997). (Stipulated Decision, License Surrender). Sacramento, CA: Board of Psychology.

In the Matter of the Accusation Against Barry G. Bachelor. (1997). Board of Psychology, State of California. Case No. W-88.

In the Matter of the Accusation Against Richard Boylon. (1994). Board of Psychology, State of California. Case No. W-14.

In the Matter of the Accusation Against Barbara Grimes. (1997). Board of Psychology, State of California. Case No. W-109.

In the Matter of the Accusation Against Judith A. Johnston. (1995). Board of Psychology, State of California. Case No. W-32.

In the Matter of the Accusation Against Larry A Nadig. (1992). Board of Psychology, State of California. Case No. D-4306.

In the Matter of the Accusation Against Leon Jerome Oziel. (1986). Board of Psychology, State of California. Case No. D-3205.

Jaffee v. Redmond, 518 U.S. 1 (1996).

James W. v. Superior Court (Goodfriend), 17 Cal.App4th 246, 21 Cal.Rptr. 169 (1993).

Jennings, F. L. (1992). Ethics in rural practice. *Psychotherapy in Private Practice, 10*, 85-104.

Keyhea v. Rushen, 178 Cal.App.3d 526, 223 Cal.Rptr. 746 (1986).

Knapp, S., & VandeCreek, L. (2003). *A Guide to the 2002 Revision of the American Psychological Association's Ethics Code*. Sarasota, FL: Professional Resource Press.

Kohlberg, L. (1981). *Essays in Moral Development, Vol. I: The Philosophy of Moral Development*. New York: Harper & Row.

Koocher, G. P., & Keith-Spiegel, P. (1998). *Ethics in Psychology: Professional Standards and Cases* (2nd ed.). New York: Oxford.

Kurpius, D., Gibson, G., Lewis, J., & Corbet, M. (1991, September). Ethical issues in supervising counseling practitioners. *Counselor Education and Supervision, 31*, 48-57.

Lakin, M. (1994). Morality in group and family therapies: Multiperson therapies and the 1992 ethics code. *Professional Psychology: Research and Practice 25*(4), 344-348.

Lazarus, A., & Zur, O. (2002). *Dual Relationships and Psychotherapy*. New York: Springer.

Lieberman, R. L., & Ebert, B. W. (1991). *Guide for Dual Relationships in Family Therapy*. Unpublished manuscript.

Lieberman, R. L., & Ebert, B. W. (1993). *Guide for Treatment of Multiple Family Members for Champus Providers*. Unpublished manuscript.

Luthman, G. L., & Kirschenbaum, M. (1974). *The Dynamic Family*. Palo Alto, CA: Science and Behavior Books.

Margolin, G. (1982, July). Ethical and legal considerations in marital and family therapy. *American Psychologist, 37*(7), 788-801.

Menendez v. Superior Court, 3 Cal.4th 435, 834 P.2d 786 (1992).

Miller, G. M., & Larrabee, M. J. (1995, June). Sexual intimacy in counselor education and supervision: A national survey. *Counselor Education and Supervision, 34*(4), 332-343.

Minuchin, S. (1974). *Families in Family Therapy*. Cambridge, MA: Harvard University Press.

Monahan, J. (1980). *Who Is the Client? The Ethics of Psychological Intervention in the Criminal Justice System*. Washington, DC: American Psychological Association.

Morrison, A. P. (1986). On projective identification in couples' groups. *International Journal of Group Psychotherapy, 36*(1), 55-73.

National Association of Social Workers (NASW). (1999). *Code of Ethics*. Washington, DC: Author.

Newman, A. (1981). Ethical issues in the supervision of psychology. *Professional Psychology: Research and Practice, 12*, 690-695.

Nugent, C. G. (1994, Winter-Spring). Blaming the victims: Silencing women sexually exploited by psychotherapists. *Journal of Mind and Behavior, 15*(1-2), 113-138.

Perkens, D. (1991). Clinical work with sex offenders in secure settings. In C. R. Hollin & K. Howells (Eds.), *Clinical Approaches to Sex Offenders and Their Victims*. New York: John Wiley.

Peterson, M. R. (1992). *At Personal Risk*. New York: W. W. Norton.

Pettifor, J. L. (1996). Ethics: Virtue and politics in the science and practice of psychology. *Canadian Psychology, 37*(1), 1-12.

Pettus v. Cole, 49 Cal.App.4th 402, 57 Cal.Rptr.2d 46 (1996).

Poliak v. Board of Psychology, 55 Cal.App4th 342, 63 Cal.Rptr.2d 866 (1997).

Pope, K. S. (1994). *Sexual Involvement With Therapists*. Washington, DC: American Psychological Association.

Pope, K. S., & Bouhoutsos, J. C. (1986). *Sexual Intimacy Between Therapists and Patients*. New York: Praeger.

Pope, K. S., & Vasquez, M. J. T. (1991). *Ethics in Psychotherapy*. New York: Random House.

Pope, K. S., & Vasquez, M. J. T. (2001). *Ethics in Psychotherapy and Counseling* (2nd ed.). San Francisco: Jossey-Bass.

Riese v. St. Mary's Hospital & Medical Center, 209 Cal.App.1303 (1987).

Rochelle v. Marine Midland Grace Trust Co., 535 F.2d 523 (9th Cir.) (1976).

Roesch, R., Zapf, P. A., Golding, S. L., & Skeem, J. J. (1999). Defining and assessing competency to stand trial. In I. B. Weiner & A. K. Hess (Eds.), *The Handbook of Forensic Psychology* (2nd ed., pp. 395-437). New York: John Wiley.

Rogers, G. L. (1996). *Benjamin Franklin's the Art of Virtue*. Eden Prairie, MN: Acorn Publishing.

Rosenthal, R. (1995). State of New Jersey v. Margaret Kelly Michaels: An overview. *Psychology, Public Policy and Law, 1*(2), 246-271.

Sagan, C. (1995). *The Demon-Haunted World*. New York: Random House.

Sales, B. D. (Ed.). (1995). Suggestibility of child witnesses – The social science amicus brief on State of New Jersey v. Margaret Kelly Michaels. *Psychology, Public Policy and Law, 1*(2), 243-520.

Satir, V. (1967). *Conjoint Family Therapy: A Guide to Theory and Technique*. Palo Alto, CA: Science and Behavior Books.

Shapiro, D. L. (1991). *Forensic Psychological Assessment: An Integrative Approach*. Boston: Allyn & Bacon.

Slimp, P. A., & Burian, B. (2003). Multiple role relationships during internship: Consequences and recommendations. In D. N. Bersoff (Ed.), *Ethical Conflicts in Psychology* (3rd ed., pp. 242-245). Washington, DC: American Psychological Association.

Solursh, D. S., Solursh, L. F., & Williams, N. R. (1993). Patient-therapist sex: "Just say no" isn't enough. *Medicine and Law, 12*(3-5), 431-438.

State v. Michaels, 625 A.2d 489 (N.J.Super.) (1993).

Swanton, C. (2003). *Virtue Ethics: A Pluralistic View.* New York: Oxford.

Syme, G. (2003). *Dual Relationships in Counseling and Psychotherapy.* Thousand Oaks, CA: Sage.

Thompson, A. (1990). *Guide to Ethical Practice in Psychotherapy.* New York: John Wiley.

United Nations. (1948). *Universal Declaration of Human Rights.* New York: Author.

United States Code Annotated, Title 11, § 10(b) (1997).

United States Code Annotated, Title 28, § 455(a) (1997).

U.S. v. Fujiwara. Moody AFB, GE (2004).

Vesper, J. H. (1995). Conflicting relationships. *American Journal of Forensic Psychology, 13*(4), 5-20.

Weissman, H. N., & DeBow, D. M. (2003). Ethical principles and professional competencies. In A. M. Goldstein (Ed.), *Handbook of Psychology: Forensic Psychology* (Vol. 11, pp. 33-53). New York: John Wiley.

Youngren, J. N., & Skorka, D. (1992). The non-therapeutic psychotherapy relationship. *Law and Psychology Review, 16,* 13-28.

SUBJECT INDEX

If You Found This Book Useful . . .

You might want to know more about our other titles.

If you would like to receive our latest catalog, please return this form:

Name: _____
(Please Print)

Address: _____

Address: _____

City/State/Zip: _____
This is ☐ home ☐ office

Telephone: (_____)_____

E-mail: _____

Fax: (_____) _____

I am a:

☐   Psychologist   ☐   Mental Health Counselor
☐   Psychiatrist   ☐   Marriage and Family Therapist
☐   Attorney   ☐   Not in Mental Health Field
☐   Clinical Social Worker   ☐   Other: _____

◆   ◆   ◆

Professional Resource Press
P.O. Box 15560
Sarasota, FL 34277-1560

Telephone: 800-443-3364
FAX: 941-343-9201
E-mail: orders@prpress.com
Website: http://www.prpress.com

Add A Colleague To Our Mailing List . . .

If you would like us to send our latest catalog to one of your colleagues, please return this form:

Name: _____
(Please Print)

Address: _____

Address: _____

City/State/Zip: _____
This is ☐ home ☐ office

Telephone: (_____)_____

E-mail: _____

Fax: (_____) _____

This person is a:

☐ Psychologist   ☐ Mental Health Counselor
☐ Psychiatrist   ☐ Marriage and Family Therapist
☐ Attorney   ☐ Not in Mental Health Field
☐ Clinical Social Worker   ☐ Other: _____

Name of person completing this form: _____

◆   ◆   ◆

Professional Resource Press
P.O. Box 15560
Sarasota, FL 34277-1560

Telephone: 800-443-3364
FAX: 941-343-9201
E-mail: orders@prpress.com
Website: http://www.prpress.com